Mendelian Randomization

Methods for Causal Inference Using Genetic Variants

CHAPMAN & HALL/CRC Interdisciplinary Statistics Series

Series editors: B.J.T. Morgan, C.K. Wikle, P.G.M. van der Heijden

For more information about this series, please visit: https://www.crcpress.com/
Chapman--HallCRC-Interdisciplinary-Statistics/book-series/CHINTSTASER

Mendelian Randomization

Methods for Causal Inference Using Genetic Variants

Second Edition

Stephen Burgess

Simon G. Thompson

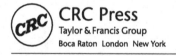

CRC Press
Taylor & Francis Group
Boca Raton London New York

CRC Press is an imprint of the
Taylor & Francis Group, an **informa** business

A CHAPMAN & HALL BOOK

First edition published 2015
by CRC Press
6000 Broken Sound Parkway NW, Suite 300, Boca Raton, FL 33487-2742

and by CRC Press
2 Park Square, Milton Park, Abingdon, Oxon, OX14 4RN

ISBN: 9780367341848 (hbk)
ISBN: 9781032019512 (pbk)
ISBN: 9780429324352 (ebk)

Typeset in CMR10
by KnowledgeWorks Global Ltd.

Contents

Preface to the second edition

The volume of research into the genetics of common diseases has exploded over the last 25 years. While many genetic variants related to various diseases have been identified, their usefulness may lie more in what they offer to our understanding of the biological mechanisms leading to disease rather than to, for example, predicting disease risk. To understand mechanisms, we need to separate the relationships of risk factors with diseases into those that are causal and those that are not. This is where Mendelian randomization can play an important role.

The technique of Mendelian randomization itself has undergone rapid development, mostly in the last 15 years, and applications now abound in medical and epidemiological journals. Its basis is that of instrumental variable analysis, which has a much longer history in statistics and particularly in econometrics. Relevant papers on Mendelian randomization are therefore dispersed across the multiple fields of genetics, epidemiology, statistics and econometrics – and increasingly bioinformatics. The intention of this book is to bring together this literature on the methods and practicalities of Mendelian randomization, especially to help those who are relatively new to this area.

In writing this book, we envisage the target audience comprising three main groups, Epidemiologists, Bioinformaticians, and Medical Statisticians, who want to perform applied Mendelian randomization analyses or understand how to interpret their results. We therefore assume a familiarity with basic epidemiological terminology, such as prospective and case-control studies, and basic statistical methods, such as linear and logistic regression. While Mendelian randomization methods can be applied in a diverse range of areas, we concentrate on applications in epidemiology, and hope that researchers in other areas will still find the content relevant.

While we have tried to ensure that this book will be accessible to a wide audience, a geneticist may baulk at the simplistic explanations of Mendelian inheritance, a statistician may yearn for a deeper level of technical exposition, and an epidemiologist may wonder why we don't just cut to the chase of how to perform the analyses. Our aim is that enough detail is given for those who need it, references are available for those who want more, and a section can simply be glossed over by those for whom it is redundant. We have also tried as far as possible to allow each chapter to be read in isolation. The price of this is that we may introduce a topic in one chapter, only to return to it in more detail in a later chapter.

While we have included relevant statistical methodology available up to the publication date of the book, our focus has been on methods and issues which are of practical relevance for applied Mendelian randomization analyses, rather than those which are of more theoretical interest, or 'cutting-edge' developments which may not stand the test of time. As such, to a research statistician, the book will provide a background to current areas of methodological debate, but it will generally not offer opinions on controversial topics which are likely to become out-of-date quickly as further investigations are performed. Where possible, sections with technical content are written in such a way that they can be omitted without interrupting the flow of the book.

A website to complement this book, as well as the authors' ongoing research on this topic, is available at www.mendelianrandomization.com. This contains chapter summaries, paper summaries, web-based applications, and software code for implementing some of the statistical techniques discussed in the book.

In preparing this second edition of this book, we substantially re-wrote and re-ordered the book to account for new developments in summarized data and two-sample Mendelian randomization, to emphasize the practical implications of methodological issues rather than their technical aspects, and to include a wider range of examples of the technique.

We would like to express our thanks to all those who commented on chapters of this book, whether in chapter or book form. We thank Frank Dudbridge, Brandon Pierce, Dylan Small, Maria Glymour, Stephen Sharp, Mary Schooling, Tom Palmer, George Davey Smith, Debbie Lawlor, John Thompson, Jack Bowden, Shaun Seaman, Lucas Tittmann, Daniel Freitag, Peter Willeit, Edmund Jones, Angela Wood, Adam Butterworth, Apostolos Gkatzionis, Andrew Grant, Verena Zuber, Eric Slob, and Dipender Gill. Further individuals commented as anonymous referees, and so we cannot thank them by name. We also thank Rob Calver, our editor, for being knowledgeable, supportive, and open to our ideas. We are grateful to the those who have allowed us to use their data in this book, either by allowing figures to be reprinted or by making summarized data publicly available, as well as to the study participants who gave their time and consent to participate in research.

In short, while we realize that we will not be able to please all of our readers all of the time, we hope that this book will enable a wide range of people to better understand what is an important, but complex and multidisciplinary, area of research.

Stephen Burgess, Simon G. Thompson

University of Cambridge, UK

First edition: August 2014.
Second edition: December 2020.

Abbreviations

2SLS	two-stage least squares
ACE	average causal effect
BMI	body mass index
CCGC	CRP CHD Genetics Collaboration
CRP	C-reactive protein
CHD	coronary heart disease
CI	confidence interval
COR	causal odds ratio
CRAN	Comprehensive R Archive Network
CRR	causal risk ratio
DNA	deoxyribonucleic acid
GMM	generalized method of moments
GWAS	genome-wide association study (or studies)
HDL	high-density lipoprotein
IL-1Ra	interleukin-1 receptor antagonist
InSIDE	instrument strength independent of direct effect
IV	instrumental variable
IVW	inverse-variance weighted
LD	linkage disequilibrium
LDL	low-density lipoprotein
LoF	loss of function
LIML	limited information maximum likelihood
Lp(a)	lipoprotein(a)
Lp-PLA$_2$	lipoprotein-associated phospholipase A$_2$
MAF	minor allele frequency
MR	Mendelian randomization
OLS	ordinary least squares
OR	odds ratio
PRESSO	pleiotropy residual sum and outlier
RAPS	robust adjusted profile score
RCT	randomized controlled trial
RSS	residual sum of squares
SE	standard error
SMM	structural mean model
SNP	single nucleotide polymorphism
ZEMPA	zero modal pleiotropy assumption

Notation

Throughout this book, we use the notation:

X	exposure: the risk factor of interest
Y	outcome
U	(sufficient) confounder of the X–Y association
G	instrumental variable
α	pleiotropic effect of a genetic variant
β	genetic association or coefficient in regression model of Y or X as function of G
β_X	genetic association with the exposure
β_Y	genetic association with the outcome
θ	coefficient in model of Y as a function of X
θ_1	causal effect of X on Y: the main parameter of interest
ρ	correlation parameter between X and Y
$\rho_{j_1 j_2}$	correlation between genetic variants j_1 and j_2
ρ_{GX}	correlation parameter between G and X
σ^2	variance parameter
ϕ^2	between-variant heterogeneity variance parameter
i	subscript indexing individuals
j	subscript indexing genetic variants
J	total number of genetic variants
k	subscript indexing exposures (multivariable Mendelian randomization)
K	total number of exposures
N	total number of individuals in sample
n	total number of cases (individuals with a disease event)
$\mathcal{N}$	normal distribution
Z	mediator on causal pathway from X to Y

For X, Y, U, and G, we follow the usual convention of using upper-case letters for random variables and lower-case letters for data values. We distinguish between parameters and their estimates by the use of hats (for example, θ is the causal effect parameter, $\hat{\theta}$ is its estimate). The standard error of an estimate is denoted $\text{se}(\hat{\theta})$.

Part I

Understanding and performing Mendelian randomization

1

Introduction and motivation

This book concerns making inferences about causal effects based on observational data using genetic variants as instrumental variables, a concept known as Mendelian randomization. In this chapter, we introduce the basic idea of Mendelian randomization, giving examples of when the approach can be used and why it may be useful. We aim in this chapter only to give a flavour of the approach; details about its conditions and requirements are reserved for later chapters. Although the examples given in this book are mainly in the context of epidemiology, Mendelian randomization can address questions in a variety of fields of study, and the majority of the material in this book is equally relevant to problems in different research areas.

1.1 Shortcomings of classical epidemiology

Epidemiology is the study of patterns of health and disease at the population level. We use the term 'classical epidemiology', meaning epidemiology without the use of genetics, to contrast with genetic epidemiology. A fundamental problem in epidemiological research, in common with other areas of social science, is the distinction between correlation and causation. If we want to address important medical questions, such as to determine disease aetiology (what is the cause of a disease?), to assess the impact of a medical or public health intervention (what would be the result of a treatment?), to inform public policy, to prioritize healthcare resources, to advise clinical practice, or to counsel on the impact of lifestyle choices, then we have to answer questions of cause and effect. The optimal way to address these questions is by appropriate study design, such as the use of prospective randomized trials.

1.1.1 Randomized trials and observational studies

The gold standard for the empirical testing of a scientific hypothesis in clinical research is a randomized controlled trial. This design involves the assignment of different treatment regimes at random to experimental units

3

(usually individuals) in a population. In its simplest form, an active treatment (for example, intervention on a risk factor) is compared against a control treatment (no intervention), and the average outcomes in each of the arms of the trial are contrasted. We will often refer to the putative causal risk factor as the 'exposure' variable. We seek to assess whether the exposure is a cause of the outcome, and estimate (if appropriate) the magnitude of the causal effect.

While randomized trials are in principle the best way of determining the causal status of a particular exposure, they have some limitations. Randomized trials are expensive and time consuming, especially when the outcome is rare or requires a long follow-up period to be observed. Additionally, in some cases, a targeted treatment which has an effect only on the exposure of interest may not be available. Moreover, many exposures cannot be randomly allocated for practical or ethical reasons. For example, in assessing the impact of drinking red wine on the risk of coronary heart disease, it would not be feasible to recruit participants to be randomly assigned to either drink or abstain from red wine over, say, a 30-year period. Alternative approaches for judging causal relationships are required.

Scientific hypotheses are often assessed using observational data. Rather than by intervening on the exposure, individuals with high and low levels of the exposure are compared. In many cases, differences between the average outcomes in the two groups have been interpreted as evidence for the causal role of the exposure. However, such a conclusion confuses correlation with causation. There are many reasons why individuals with elevated levels of the exposure may have greater average outcome levels, without the exposure being a causal agent.

Interpreting an association between an exposure and a disease outcome in observational data as a causal relationship relies on untestable and usually implausible assumptions, such as the absence of unmeasured confounding (see Chapter 2) and of reverse causation. This has led to several high-profile cases where an exposure has been widely promoted as an important factor in disease prevention based on observational data, only to be later discredited when evidence from randomized trials did not support a causal interpretation [Taubes and Mann, 1995]. For example, observational studies reported a strong inverse association between vitamin C and risk of coronary heart disease, which did not attenuate on adjustment for a variety of alternative risk factors [Khaw et al., 2001]. However, experimental data results obtained from randomized trials showed a non-significant association in the opposite direction [Collins et al., 2002]. The confidence interval for the observational association did not include the randomized trial estimate [Davey Smith and Ebrahim, 2003]. Similar stories apply to the observational and experimental associations between β-carotene and smoking-related cancers [Peto et al., 1981; Hennekens et al., 1996], and between vitamin E and coronary heart disease [Hooper et al., 2001]. More worrying is the history of hormone-replacement therapy, which was previously advocated as being beneficial for the reduction of breast cancer and cardiovascular mortality on the basis of observational data, but was subsequently shown to increase mortality in randomized trials [Rossouw et al., 2002; Beral et al., 2003]. More reliable approaches are therefore needed for assessing causal relationships using observational data. Mendelian randomization is one such approach.

1.2   The rise of genetic epidemiology

Genetic epidemiology is the study of the role of genetic factors in health and disease for populations. We sketch the history and development of genetic epidemiology, indicating why it is an important area of epidemiological and scientific research.

1.2.1   Historical background

Although the inheritance of characteristics from one generation to the next has been observed for millennia, the mechanism for inheritance was long unknown. When Charles Darwin first proposed his theory of evolution in 1859, one of its major problems was the lack of an underlying mechanism for heredity [Darwin, 1871]. Gregor Mendel in 1866 proposed two laws of inheritance: the law of segregation, that when any individual produces gametes (sex cells), the two copies of a gene separate so that each gamete receives only one copy; and the law of independent assortment, that 'unlinked or distantly linked segregating gene pairs assort independently at meiosis [cell division]' [Mendel, 1866]. These laws are summarized by the term 'Mendelian inheritance', and it is this which gives Mendelian randomization its name [Davey Smith and Ebrahim, 2003]. The two areas of evolution and Mendelian inheritance were brought together through the 1910s–30s in the 'modern evolutionary synthesis', by amongst others Ronald Fisher, who helped to develop population genetics [Fisher, 1918]. A direct connection between genetics and disease was established by Linus Pauling in 1949, who linked a specific genetic mutation in patients with sickle-cell anaemia to a change in the haemoglobin of the red blood cells [Pauling et al., 1949]. The discovery of the structure of deoxyribonucleic acid (DNA) in 1953 gave rise to the birth of molecular biology, which led to greater understanding of the genetic code [Watson and Crick, 1953]. The Human Genome Project was established in 1990, leading to the publication of the entirety of the human genetic code by the early 2000s [Roberts et al., 2001; McPherson et al., 2001]. Recently, technological advances have reduced the cost of DNA sequencing to the level where it is now economically viable to measure genetic information for a large number of individuals [Shendure and Ji, 2008].

1.2.2 Genetics and disease

As the knowledge of the human genome has developed, the search for genetic determinants of disease has expanded from monogenic disorders (disorders which are due to a single mutated gene, such as sickle-cell anaemia), to polygenic and multifactorial disorders, where the burden of disease risk is not due to a single gene, but to multiple genes combined with lifestyle and environmental factors. These diseases, such as cancers, diabetes, and coronary heart disease, tend to cluster within families, but also depend on modifiable risk factors, such as diet and blood pressure. Several genetic factors have been found which relate to these diseases, especially through the increased use of genome-wide association studies (GWAS), in which the associations of hundreds of thousands or even millions of genetic variants with a disease outcome are tested. In some cases, these discoveries have added to the scientific understanding of disease processes and the ability to predict disease risk for individuals. Nevertheless, they are of limited immediate interest from a clinical perspective, as an individual's genome cannot currently be changed. However, genetic discoveries provide opportunities for Mendelian randomization: a technique for using genetic data to assess and estimate causal effects of modifiable non-genetic exposures based on observational data.

1.3 Motivating example: The inflammation hypothesis

We introduce the approach of Mendelian randomization using an example. The inflammation hypothesis is an important question in the understanding of cardiovascular disease. Inflammation is one of the body's response mechanisms to a harmful stimulus. It is characterized by redness, swelling, heat, pain, and loss of function in the affected body area. Cases can be divided into acute inflammation, which refers to the initial response of the body, and chronic inflammation, which refers to more prolonged changes. Examples of conditions classified as inflammation include appendicitis, chilblains, and arthritis.

Cardiovascular disease is a term covering a range of diseases including coronary heart disease (in particular myocardial infarction or a 'heart attack') and stroke. It is currently the biggest cause of death worldwide. The inflammation hypothesis states that there is some aspect of the inflammation response mechanism which leads to cardiovascular disease events, and that intervening on this pathway will reduce the risk of cardiovascular disease.

1.3.1 C-reactive protein and coronary heart disease

As part of the inflammation process, several chemicals are produced by the body, known as (positive) acute-phase proteins. These represent the body's first line of defence against infection and injury. There has been particular interest in one of these, C-reactive protein (CRP), and the role of elevated levels of CRP in the risk of coronary heart disease (CHD). It is known that CRP is observationally associated with the risk of CHD [Kaptoge et al., 2010], but, prior to robust Mendelian randomization studies, it was not known whether this association was causal [Danesh and Pepys, 2009]. The specific question in this example (a small part of the wider inflammation hypothesis) is whether long-term elevated levels of CRP lead to greater risk of CHD.

1.3.2   Alternative explanations for association

In our example, there are many factors that increase both levels of CRP and the risk of CHD. These factors, known as confounders, may be measured and accounted for by statistical analysis, for instance multivariable regression. However, it is not possible to know whether all such factors have been identified. Also, CRP levels increase in response to sub-clinical disease, giving the possibility that the observed association is due to reverse causation.

One of the potential confounders of particular interest is fibrinogen, a soluble blood plasma glycoprotein, which enables blood-clotting. It is also part of the inflammation pathway. Although CRP is observationally positively associated with CHD risk, this association was shown to reduce on adjustment for various conventional risk factors (such as age, sex, body mass index, and diabetes status), and to attenuate to near null on further adjustment for fibrinogen [Kaptoge et al., 2010]. It is important to assess whether elevated levels of CRP are causally related to changes in fibrinogen, since if so conditioning the CRP–CHD association on fibrinogen would represent an over-adjustment, which would attenuate a true causal effect.

1.3.3   Instrumental variables

To address the problems of confounding and reverse causation in conventional epidemiology, we introduce the concept of an instrumental variable. An instrumental variable is a measurable quantity (a variable) which is associated with the exposure of interest, but not associated with any other competing risk factor that is a confounder for the outcome. Neither does it influence the outcome directly, but only potentially indirectly via the hypothesized causal pathway through the exposure under investigation. A potential example of an instrumental variable for health outcomes is geographic location. We imagine that two neighbouring regions have different policies on how to treat patients, and assume that patients who live on one side of the border are similar in all respects to those on the other side of the border, except that they receive different treatment regimes. By comparing these groups of patients, geographic location acts like the random allocation to treatment assignment in a randomized controlled trial, influencing the exposure of interest without being associated with competing risk factors. It therefore is an instrumental variable, and gives rise to a natural experiment in the population, from which causal inferences can be obtained. Other plausible non-genetic instrumental variables include government policy changes (for example, the introduction of a smoking ban in public places, or an increase in cigarette tax, which might decrease cigarette smoking prevalence without changing other variables) and physician prescribing preference (for example, the treatment a doctor chose to prescribe to the previous patient, which will be representative of the doctor's preferred treatment, but should not be affected by the current patient's personal characteristics or case history).

1.3.4   Genetic variants as instrumental variables

A genetic variant is a section of genetic code that differs between individuals. In Mendelian randomization, genetic variants are used as instrumental variables. Individuals in a population can be divided into subgroups based on their genetic variants. On the assumption that the genetic variants can be treated as if they have been randomly distributed in the population (by this, we mean that they are independent of environmental and other variables), then these genetic subgroups do not systematically differ with respect to any of these variables. Additionally, as the genetic code for each individual is determined before birth, there is no way that a variable measured in a mature individual can causally precede a genetic variant. Returning to our example, if we can find a suitable genetic variant (or variants) associated with CRP levels, then we can compare the genetically defined subgroup of individuals with lower average levels of CRP to the subgroup with higher average levels of CRP. In effect, we are exploiting a natural experiment in the population, whereby nature has randomly given some individuals a genetic 'treatment' which increases their CRP levels. If individuals with a genetic variant that is associated with elevated average levels of CRP and satisfies the instrumental variable assumptions exhibit greater incidence of CHD, then we can conclude that CRP is a causal risk factor for CHD, and that lowering CRP is likely to lead to reductions in CHD rates. Under further assumptions about the statistical model for the relationship between CRP and CHD risk, a causal parameter can be estimated. Although Mendelian randomization uses genetic variants to answer inferential questions, these are not questions about genetics, but rather about modifiable exposures, such as CRP, and their causal effects on outcomes (usually disease outcomes).

1.3.5   Violations of instrumental variable assumptions

It is impossible to test whether there is a causal relationship between two variables on the basis of observational data alone. All empirical methods for making causal claims by necessity rely on untestable assumptions.

Instrumental variable methods are no exception. Taking the example of Section 1.3.3, if geographic location is associated with other factors, such as socioeconomic status, then the assumption that the distribution of the outcome would be the same for both populations under each policy regime would be violated. Or if the genetic variant(s) associated with CRP levels used in a Mendelian randomization analysis were also independently associated with, say, blood pressure, the comparison of genetic subgroups would not be a valid test for the causal hypothesis that CRP affects CHD risk. The validity of the instrumental variable assumptions is crucial to the interpretation of a Mendelian randomization investigation and is discussed at length in later chapters.

1.4 Other examples of Mendelian randomization

Although the initial applications of Mendelian randomization were in the field of epidemiology [Youngman et al., 2000], the use of genetic instrumental variables is becoming widespread in a number of different fields. A systematic review of applied Mendelian randomization studies was published in 2010 [Bochud and Rousson, 2010]. A list of the exposures and outcomes of some causal relationships which have been assessed using Mendelian randomization is given in Table 1.1. The list includes examples with a wide range of exposure and outcome variables in epidemiology, psychology, and social science: the only limitation in the use of Mendelian randomization to assess the causal effect of an exposure on an outcome is the availability of a suitable genetic variant to use as the instrumental variable.

The reasons to use Mendelian randomization outside of epidemiology are similar to those in epidemiology. In many fields, randomized experiments are difficult to perform and instrumental variable techniques represent one of the few ways of assessing causal relationships in the absence of complete knowledge of confounders.

1.5 Overview of book

Although there has been much research into the use of instrumental variables in econometrics and epidemiology since they were first proposed [Wright, 1928], several barriers existed in applying this to the context of Mendelian randomization. These include differences in terminology, where the same concept is referred to in various disciplines by different names, and differences in theoretical concepts, particularly relating to the definition and

Category	Exposure	Outcome	Reference
Biomarker	Fibrinogen	CHD	[1]
	CRP	CIMT	[2]
	SHBG	Type 2 diabetes	[3]
	Lipoprotein(a)	Myocardial infarction	[4–5]
	Homocysteine	Stroke	[6]
	Lipids	AMD	[7]
	Inflammatory markers	Depression	[8]
	Serum urate	CHD	[9]
	Serum calcium	CHD	[10]
Complex risk factor	BMI	Breast cancer	[11]
	Blood pressure	Valvular heart disease	[12]
	Resting heart rate	CHD	[13]
	Education	Alzheimer's disease	[14]
	Myopia	Educational attainment	[15]
	Age at puberty	Asthma	[16]
Dietary / lifestyle factor	Vitamin D	Multiple sclerosis	[17]
	Cannabis initiation	Schizophrenia	[18]
	Alcohol intake	Blood pressure	[19]
	Caffeine intake	Stillbirth	[20]
	Milk intake	Metabolic syndrome	[21]
	Foetal alcohol	IQ	[22]

TABLE 1.1

Examples of causal relationships assessed by Mendelian randomization in applied research.

Abbreviations:
AMD = age-related macular degeneration, BMI = body mass index, CHD = coronary heart disease, CIMT = carotid intima-media thickness, CRP = C-reactive protein, IQ = intelligence quotient, SHBG = sex hormone-binding globulin.

References:
1. Keavney et al., 2006
2. Kivimäki et al., 2008
3. Ding et al., 2009
4. Kamstrup et al., 2009
5. Clarke et al., 2009
6. Casas et al., 2005
7. Burgess and Davey Smith, 2017
8. Khandaker et al., 2020
9. White et al., 2015
10. Larsson et al., 2017a
11. Guo et al., 2017
12. Nazarzadeh et al., 2019
13. Eppinga et al., 2016
14. Larsson et al., 2017b
15. Mountjoy et al., 2018
16. Minelli et al., 2018
17. Mokry et al., 2015
18. Gage et al., 2017
19. Chen et al., 2008
20. Bech et al., 2006
21. Almon et al., 2010
22. Lewis et al., 2012.

interpretation of causal relationships. Additionally, several methodological issues have been raised by the use of genetic variants as instrumental variables that had not previously been considered in the instrumental variables literature, and required (and still require) methodological development. A major motivation in writing this book is to provide an accessible resource to those coming from different academic disciplines to understand issues relevant to the use of genetic variants as instrumental variables, particularly for those wanting to undertake and interpret Mendelian randomization analyses.

1.5.1 Structure

This book is divided into three parts. The first part, comprising Chapters 1 to 6, is titled 'Understanding and performing Mendelian randomization'. This part contains the essential information for a practitioner interested in Mendelian randomization (Chapters 1 and 2), including definitions of causal effects and instrumental variables (Chapter 3), and methods for the estimation of causal effects using individual-level data (Chapter 4) and summarized data (Chapter 5). Also addressed is the question of how to interpret a Mendelian randomization estimate, and how it may compare to the effect of an intervention on the exposure of interest in practice (Chapter 6). These sections should be fully accessible to most epidemiologists and other researchers with some training in quantitative data analysis, but should not need a mathematical background to understand. While we have provided technical details, these are not essential to the understanding of the concepts, and can generally be glossed over by the less technical reader.

The second part, comprising Chapters 7 to 10, is titled 'Advanced methods for Mendelian randomization'. In many cases, Mendelian randomization analyses using different genetic variants as instrumental variables lead to causal estimates which differ to the extent that they are not mutually compatible. This typically means that not all of those variants satisfy the instrumental variable assumptions. Robust methods have been developed that are able to consistently estimate a causal parameter under weaker assumptions. In Chapter 7, we describe all commonly used robust methods. In Chapter 8, we present matters concerning the behaviour of instrumental variable estimates, such as their statistical properties and potential sources of bias. In Chapter 9, we consider extensions to the basic Mendelian randomization paradigm. Chapter 10 provides a practical overview of how to perform a Mendelian randomization investigation, from the motivation and conceptualization of the research question, through to the interpretation of results. Although some of the details in this part of the book require a greater depth of mathematical understanding, each concept is introduced and described using non-technical language as far as possible.

Finally in Chapter 11, we conclude by discussing current and future directions for research involving Mendelian randomization.

1.6 Summary

Distinguishing between a factor which is merely associated with an outcome and one which has a causal effect on the outcome is problematic outside of the context of a randomized controlled trial. Instrumental variables provide a way of assessing causal relationships in observational data, and Mendelian randomization is the use of genetic variants as instrumental variables.

In the next chapter, we provide more detail of what Mendelian randomization is, and when and why it may be useful.

2

What is Mendelian randomization?

In this chapter, we illustrate in more depth the conceptual framework and motivation for Mendelian randomization, explaining how Mendelian randomization offers opportunities to address some of the problems of conventional epidemiology. We describe the specific characteristics of genetic data which give rise to the Mendelian randomization approach, and provide a classification of Mendelian randomization investigations.

2.1 What is Mendelian randomization?

Mendelian randomization is the use of genetic variants in non-experimental data to make inferences about the causal effect of an exposure on an outcome. We use the word 'exposure' throughout this book to refer to the putative causal risk factor. It can be a biomarker, an anthropometric measure, a dietary or lifestyle factor, or any other risk factor that may affect the outcome. Usually the outcome is disease, although there is no methodological restriction as to what outcomes can be considered. Non-experimental data encompass all observational studies, including cross-sectional and longitudinal, cohort, and case-control designs – any study where there is no intervention applied by the researcher.

2.1.1 Motivation

A foundational aim of epidemiological research is the estimation of the impact on an outcome of changing an exposure. This is known as the causal effect of the exposure on the outcome. It typically differs from the observational association between the exposure and outcome, due to factors such as confounding. Correlation between the exposure and the outcome cannot be reliably interpreted as evidence of a causal relationship. For example, those who drink red wine regularly have a lower incidence of heart disease than those who do not drink red wine. But socio-economic status is a common predictor of both wine consumption and better coronary health, and so it may be that socio-economic status rather than wine consumption underlies the reduction in heart disease risk. Observational associations may also arise as a result of reverse causation. For example, those who regularly take headache tablets are likely to have more headaches than those who do not, but taking headache tablets is unlikely to be a cause of the increased incidence of headaches. Another example is vitamin D levels, which may decrease in individuals who are ill and therefore do not go outside, rather than vitamin D being a cause of illness.

The idea of Mendelian randomization is to find a genetic variant (or variants) associated with the exposure, but not associated with any other risk factor which affects the outcome, and that does not directly affect the outcome. This means that any association of the genetic variant with the outcome must come via the variant's association with the exposure, and therefore implies a causal effect of the exposure on the outcome. Such a genetic variant would satisfy the assumptions of an instrumental variable (IV) [Greenland, 2000a; Sussman et al., 2010]. As the theory of IVs was initially developed in the field of econometrics, a number of terms commonly used in the IV literature derive from this field and are not always well understood by medical statisticians or epidemiologists. Table 2.1 is a glossary of terms which are used in each field.

2.1.2 Instrumental variables

A technical definition of Mendelian randomization is 'instrumental variable analysis using genetic instruments' [Wehby et al., 2008]. In Mendelian randomization, genetic variants are used as IVs for assessing the causal effect of the exposure on the outcome [Thomas and Conti, 2004].

The fundamental conditions for a genetic variant to satisfy to be an IV are summarized as:

i. the variant is associated with the exposure,

ii. the variant is not associated with the outcome via a confounding pathway,

iii. the variant does not affect the outcome directly, only possibly indirectly via the exposure.

Although Mendelian randomization analyses may involve a single genetic variant, multiple variants can be used either as separate IVs or combined into a single IV. More detail on the IV assumptions, which are key to the validity of Mendelian randomization investigations, is given in Chapter 3.

2.1.3 Confounding and endogeneity

One of the reasons why there may be a correlation between the exposure and outcome in an observational study is confounding, or the related concept, endogeneity of the exposure.

Econometrics term	Epidemiological term	Notes
Endogenous / endogeneity Exogenous / exogeneity	Confounded / confounding Unconfounded / no confounding	A variable is confounded / endogenous in a regression model if it is correlated with the error term, meaning that the regression coefficient is a biased estimate of the causal effect. A variable is unconfounded / exogenous if it is not correlated with the error term (see Section 2.1.3).
Outcome	Outcome	Denoted Y in this text.
Endogenous regressor	Exposure	Denoted X in this text; the causal effect of X on Y cannot be estimated by simple regression of Y on X if there is unmeasured confounding.
Instrumental variable / excluded instrument	Instrumental variable / instrument	Denoted G in this text; the instrument is called 'excluded' because it is not included in the second-stage of the two-stage regression method often used for calculating IV estimates.
Included regressor	Measured covariate	A covariate that is included in a model, such as a multivariable regression.
OLS	Least-squares regression	OLS stands for ordinary least squares. The OLS estimate is a measure of the observational association, as opposed to the IV estimate, which is a measure of the causal effect.
Concentrate out	Profile out	To exclude a nuisance parameter from an equation by forming a profile likelihood with its maximum likelihood estimate given the other variables.
Overidentification	Heterogeneity	An overidentification / heterogeneity test assesses whether different IVs have similar causal estimates.
Panel data	Longitudinal data	Data on items at multiple timepoints.

TABLE 2.1

A summary of instrumental variable terms used in the fields of econometrics and epidemiology.

Confounding is defined as the presence of inherent differences between groups with different levels of the exposure [Greenland and Robins, 1986]. It is often considered to result from the distribution of particular variables in the population, known as confounders. A confounder is a variable which is a common cause of both the exposure and the outcome. When confounders are recognized, measured, and adjusted for (for example, in multivariable regression), the remaining association between the exposure and outcome will often still be a biased estimate of the causal effect, due to the existence of unknown or unmeasured confounders or imprecision in measured confounders. Confounding not adjusted for in an analysis is termed 'residual confounding'.

Endogeneity means that there is a correlation between the regressor and the error term in a regression model. The words 'exogenous' and 'endogenous' are rarely used in epidemiology (see Table 2.1), but the terms have rigorous definitions that are useful in understanding confounding. Endogeneity literally means 'coming from within'. The opposite of endogenous is exogenous; an exogenous variable 'comes from outside' of the regression model. The term endogeneity encompasses confounding, but also includes phenomena that are traditionally thought of as separate from confounding, such as differential measurement error and reverse causation. If the exposure in a model is endogenous in a regression model, then the regression coefficient for the exposure will be biased for the causal effect. An IV can be understood as an exogenous variable, associated with an endogenous exposure, which is used to estimate the average difference in the outcome at different average values of the exposure when all other factors are on average equal [Martens et al., 2006]. Under the consistency assumption, this unconfounded estimate can be interpreted as a causal effect. The consistency assumption states that the same value of the outcome is obtained when the exposure is observed to take a certain value as when the exposure is set to take the same value (see Section 3.3).

Mendelian randomization has also been named 'Mendelian deconfounding' [Tobin et al., 2004] as it aims to give estimates of a causal effect free from biases due to confounding. The correlations between risk factors make it impossible in an observational study to find groups in the population that differ in one variable while all others remain equal, as differences in one factor will typically be accompanied by differences in other factors. While we can measure individual confounders and adjust for them in our analysis, we can never be certain that all confounders have been identified or measured precisely, leading to residual confounding. Additionally, if we adjust for a variable that lies on the true causal pathway between the exposure of interest and outcome (a mediator), this represents an over-adjustment and attenuates the estimate of the causal effect [Christenfeld et al., 2004]. By finding a genetic variant which satisfies the IV assumptions, we can estimate the unconfounded association between the exposure and the outcome even without complete knowledge of all confounders.

2.1.4 Analogy with a randomized controlled trial

Mendelian randomization is analogous to a randomized controlled trial (RCT) [Nitsch et al., 2006]. An RCT, considered to provide the gold standard of medical evidence, involves dividing a set of individuals into two or more subgroups in a random way. These subgroups are each given different treatments. Randomization is preferred over any other assignment to subgroups as all possible confounders, known and unknown, are on average balanced between the subgroups.

In Mendelian randomization, we use a genetic variant to form subgroups analogous to those in an RCT, as shown in Figure 2.1. From the IV assumptions (Section 2.1.2), these subgroups differ systematically in the exposure, but not in any other factor except for those causally 'downstream' of the exposure. A difference in the average outcome between these subgroups would therefore indicate a causal effect of the exposure on the outcome [Hernán and Robins, 2006]. Inferring a causal effect of the exposure on the outcome from an association between the genetic variant and the outcome is analogous to inferring an intention-to-treat effect from an association between randomization and the outcome in an RCT. If the RCT is properly blinded, then treatment assignment is independent of all causes of the outcome, and the only way that treatment assignment can influence the outcome is via the treatment itself. Hence treatment assignment in an RCT is an IV. Any association between treatment assignment and the outcome must be due to the causal effect of the treatment.

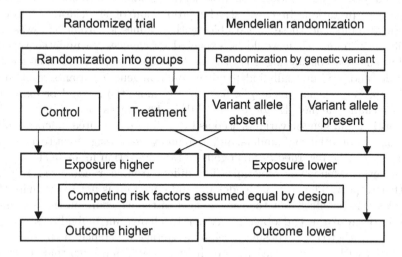

FIGURE 2.1

Comparison of a randomized controlled trial and Mendelian randomization.

Genetic variants for an individual are inherited from their parents, and so their assignment is not entirely random. For example, if neither of an individual's parents carry a particular genetic mutation, the individual will not carry that mutation. Nonetheless, under fairly realistic conditions the distribution of genetic variants in the population can be treated as random with respect to confounders. Sufficient assumptions for a variant to be randomly distributed are random mating and lack of selection effects relating to the variant of interest. Indeed, even in the absence of Mendel's laws of inheritance, random mating would ensure that genetic variants are distributed independently of confounders. Considerable departures from the random mating assumptions which may invalidate the use of a genetic variant can be assessed by performing a test of Hardy–Weinberg equilibrium, to see if the frequency of heterozygotes and homozygotes (see Section 2.3) in the population is in line with what is expected. A variable which is distributed 'as if' being randomly assigned despite the lack of true randomness in the assignment is known as quasi-randomized. Most natural experiments rely on quasi-randomization rather than the strict randomization of experimental units.

While there will be some departures from the random mating assumption, studies have shown that common genetic variants appear to be distributed independently of potential confounders in the population, at least in a Western European context. An observational study showed that linear regression gave a p-value less than 0.01 in 45% of 4560 associations between all pairs of 96 non-genetic variables [Davey Smith et al., 2007]. This suggests that many observed associations between environmental variables may not have a true causal interpretation. In contrast, the proportion of associations between genetic variants and these 96 variables with p-values less than 0.01 was not significantly higher than would be expected by chance. An updated version of this analysis considering 1 171 764 associations between 121 non-genetic variables and 9684 mutually independent common genetic variants resulted in 60 136 (5.1%) associations at $p < 0.05$, barely more than would be expected due to chance alone [Taylor et al., 2017]. This gives plausibility to the assumption that genetic variants used as IVs will be distributed independently from many potential confounders, and so in many cases assignment to a genetic subgroup can be regarded as analogous to randomization in an RCT.

However, Mendelian randomization differs from a randomized trial in another respect. The aim of Mendelian randomization is not to estimate the size of a genetic effect, but the causal effect of the exposure on the outcome. This is because the end objective is not to change an individual's genetic code, but rather their exposure level. The average difference in the outcome associated with a genetic variant may differ in magnitude from that resulting from an intervention in the exposure (see Chapter 6). Additionally, even if the association of a genetic variant with the outcome is small in magnitude, the population attributable risk of the exposure is not necessarily low, as the exposure may vary to a considerably larger extent than that which can be explained by the variant. It may be possible to change the exposure by a greater amount than the mean difference in the exposure between genetic subgroups. For example, the effect of statin drug use on low-density lipoprotein cholesterol levels is several times larger than the association of low-density lipoprotein cholesterol levels with variants in the *HMGCR* gene, and consequently the potential effect on subsequent outcomes is greater than the genetic associations with those outcomes.

2.2 Why use Mendelian randomization?

Although the main reason to use Mendelian randomization is to avoid the problem of residual confounding, there are additional reasons for using Mendelian randomization in specific contexts: with case-control data and with exposures that are difficult to measure.

2.2.1 Reverse causation and case-control studies

Reverse causation occurs when an association between the exposure and the outcome is not due to the exposure causing a change in the outcome, but the outcome causing a change in the exposure. This could happen if the exposure increased in response to pre-clinical disease, for example, from cancer before it becomes clinically apparent or from atherosclerosis prior to clinical manifestations of coronary heart disease. As the genotype of an individual is determined at conception and cannot be changed, there is no possibility of reverse causation by which a disease changes an individual's genotype.

For this reason, Mendelian randomization has great strengths in a retrospective setting where genetic variants are measured after the disease outcome, such as in a case-control study. Many exposures of interest cannot be reliably measured in cases, that is in individuals who have already experienced an outcome event, as the disease event may distort the measurement. In this situation, the genetic variant can be used as a proxy for the exposure, and the genetic association with the outcome can be assessed retrospectively. As the genotype of an individual can be measured in diseased individuals, reliable causal inferences can be obtained using Mendelian randomization in a case-control setting.

2.2.2 Exposures that are expensive or difficult to measure

Mendelian randomization can be a useful technique when the exposure of interest is expensive or difficult to measure. For example, gold-standard assays for biomarkers such as water-soluble vitamins may cost too much to be affordable for a large sample, or measurement of fasting blood glucose, which requires overnight fasting, may be impractical. If the genetic variant is associated with the exposure (this can be verified in a subsample or a separate dataset) and is a valid IV for the exposure, a causal relationship between the exposure and the outcome can be inferred from an association between the genetic variant and the outcome even in the absence of exposure measurements.

Additionally, in large samples instrumental variable estimates do not attenuate due to classical measurement error (including within-individual variation) in the exposure [Pierce and VanderWeele, 2012]. This contrasts with classical observational studies, in which measurement error in the exposure usually leads to the attenuation of regression coefficients towards the null (known as regression dilution bias) [Frost and Thompson, 2000].

A further example is where the risk factor is not only difficult to measure, but also difficult to define. For example, a variant in the *IL6R* gene region that is associated with serum interleukin-6 concentrations (as well as levels of downstream inflammatory markers, including C-reactive protein and fibrinogen) was shown to be associated with coronary heart disease (CHD) risk [Swerdlow et al., 2012]. However, from knowledge about the functional role of the variant, the causal effect assessed is not thought to operate through elevated serum interleukin-6 concentrations, but rather through changes in signalling in interleukin-6 receptor pathways. This is a cellular phenotype which varies over time, and so a representative measurement for an individual is not straightforward to define. However, as the genetic variant can be measured, the causal role of interleukin-6 receptor-related pathways on CHD risk can be assessed by Mendelian randomization [Sarwar et al., 2012].

2.3   A brief overview of genetics

In order to understand Mendelian randomization, it is necessary to have at least a cursory understanding of genetics. We here provide a brief overview of genetics, only covering the information necessary to understand Mendelian randomization. A glossary of genetic terminology, adapted from a Mendelian randomization review paper [Lawlor et al., 2008] is provided in Table 2.2. Further information on genetic terminology related to Mendelian randomization can be found in other papers [Davey Smith and Ebrahim, 2003; Sheehan et al., 2008].

2.3.1   Reading the genetic code

The genetic information (or genome) of many living organisms consists of long strings of genetic code in the form of DNA (deoxyribonucleic acid), the molecule that encodes life, packaged up into chromosomes. Humans have

- *Alleles* are the variant forms of a single nucleotide polymorphism (SNP). For a *biallelic SNP*, there are two possible alleles: the more common allele is called the *major allele* or *wildtype allele*, and the less common allele is the *minor allele* or *variant allele*.
- A *chromosome* carries a collection of genes located on a long string of DNA. Humans have 22 pairs of autosomal (non-sex) chromosomes and 1 pair of sex chromosomes.
- A *copy number variant* (or *variation*) is a (possibly) repeating section of DNA where the number of copies of the section varies between individuals.
- *DNA* (deoxyribonucleic acid) is a molecule that contains the genetic instructions needed to construct other components of cells, including proteins and ribonucleic acid (RNA) molecules. DNA has four nucleotide bases labelled A, T, C, and G.
- A *gene* is a section of a chromosome comprising DNA which encodes information relevant to the function of an organism.
- The *genotype* of an individual at a particular locus refers to the two alleles at that locus. If the alleles are the same, the genotype is *homozygous*; if different, *heterozygous*.
- A *genome-wide association study* (GWAS) is an observational study of set of genetic variants from across the genome to find variants associated with a trait. Typically only associations achieving a strict level of statistical significance (such as $p < 5 \times 10^{-8}$) are considered to be *genome-wide significant*.
- A *haplotype* describes a particular combination of alleles from linked loci found on a single chromosome.
- *Linkage disequilibrium* (LD) is the correlation between allelic states at different loci within the population typically arising due to physical proximity of the loci. The term LD describes a state that represents a departure from the hypothetical situation in which all loci exhibit complete independence (*linkage equilibrium*).
- A *locus* (plural: *loci*) is the position in a DNA sequence and can be a single position (such as the location of a SNP), a region of DNA sequence, or a whole gene.
- A *phenotype* is an observable characteristic or trait. The term phenotype (or *phenotypic*) is often used in contrast to genotype (or genotypic) to describe the exposure or another potential risk factor trait.
- *Pleiotropy* is the potential for genes or genetic variants to have more than one independent phenotypic effect.
- *Polymorphism* is the existence of two or more variants at a locus. The term polymorphism is usually restricted to moderately common genetic variants, with at least two alleles having frequencies of greater than 1% in the population. A less common variant allele is called a mutation.
- *Single nucleotide polymorphisms* (SNPs) are genetic variations in which one base in the DNA is altered, for example, a C instead of an T.

TABLE 2.2
A glossary of genetic terminology, adapted from Lawlor et al. [2008].

23 pairs of chromosomes, with one chromosome in each of the pairs coming from the mother and one from the father. Chromosomes contain genes, which are locatable regions of the genetic code that encode a unit of heritable information. Not all of the genetic sequence falls into a gene region, and much of the chromosome consists of intermediate genetic material known as non-coding DNA.

A single chromosome has two strands, each consisting of a sequence of nucleotide bases which can represented by letters. There are four possible nucleotide bases (adenine, thymine, cytosine, and guanine) represented by the letters A, T, C, and G. These nucleotide bases pair up in such a way that the strands contain complementary sequences. Wherever the first strand has A, the other will have T – and vice versa. Wherever the first strand has C, the other will have G – and vice versa. In this way, each of the strands contains the same information, and so only one of the strands is considered. Suppose that a chromosome at a given locus (position) in the DNA sequence on one of its strands reads:

...ATTACGC<u>T</u>TCCGAGCTTCCGCAG...

and that same locus on the paired chromosome reads:

...ATTACGC<u>C</u>TCCGAGCTTCCGCAG...

The underlined nucleotide represents a nucleotide at a particular locus that is polymorphic: it exists in various forms. All individuals contain many genetic mutations, where the DNA code has changed from that generally seen in the population. A single nucleotide polymorphism (SNP) is a mutation where a single nucleotide base at a particular locus has been replaced with a different nucleotide. The different possible nucleotides which may appear at each locus are known as alleles. For example, at the highlighted locus above, one chromosome has the letter T, and the other has the letter C: so T and C are alleles of this particular SNP. If these are the only two possibilities, this is a biallelic SNP; triallelic and quadrallelic SNPs are less common, but have also been observed.

For a biallelic SNP, it is conventional to denote the more common allele, known as the wildtype or major allele, by an upper case letter (for example, A) and the less common allele, the variant or minor allele, by a lower case letter (for example, a). The choice of letter is arbitrary; there is no connection between the letter A commonly used for the first variant considered, and the nucleotide base adenine represented by letter A. The proportion of minor alleles in a population for a given SNP is called the 'minor allele frequency'. Although some genetic mutations seem to be specific to particular individuals, others are more widespread, showing up in a substantial proportion of the population. SNPs occur on average about once in every 300 nucleotides along the genome, and extensive catalogues of SNPs have been compiled.

As people have two copies of each chromosome (one from each parent), individuals can be categorized for each biallelic SNP into three possible subgroups corresponding to their combination of alleles (their genotype). These subgroups are the major homozygotes (AA), heterozygotes (Aa) and minor homozygotes (aa). We can denote these subgroups as 0, 1, and 2, corresponding to the number of minor alleles for that SNP. However, there is no reason to count the number of minor alleles rather than the number of major alleles; subgroups based on the same SNP could be denoted as 2, 1, and 0. The allele that is counted is generally called the 'effect allele'. However, terminology varies between sources; in some publications, the term 'reference allele' refers to the effect allele, and in other publications, the same term refers to the non-effect allele.

For a more complicated genetic variant, such as a triallelic SNP where there are three possible alleles at one locus, there is no natural ordering of the six possible subgroups given by the SNP. A further type of polymorphism is an indel (a combination of the words 'insertion' and 'deletion'). The simplest form of indel is a single base pair insertion, meaning that a chromosome may have an additional letter in its genetic code sequence at a particular locus. Again, an indel can divide individuals into subgroups denoted as 0, 1, and 2, referring to the number of insertions (or deletions) in an individual's two chromosomes at that locus.

When multiple SNPs on a single chromosome are considered, the combination of alleles on each of the chromosomes is known as a haplotype. For example, if an individual has one chromosome reading:

...GCACC**T**TAC...GTA**G**AATC...TCAACTG**T**CAT

and the other reading:

...GCACC**G**TAC...GTA**A**AATC...TCAACTG**T**CAT

then the individual is a heterozygote for the first two SNPs, and a homozygote for the final SNP. The haplotypes are TGT and GAT. One of these haplotypes is inherited from each of the individual's parents. As a haplotype is a series of alleles on the same chromosome, haplotype patterns, especially for SNPs that are physically close together, are often inherited together. This means that genetic variants are not always independently distributed.

Other patterns of genetic variation can also be used as IVs, such as copy number variations where a section of genetic material is repeated a variable number of times. Generally, throughout this book we shall assume that IVs are biallelic SNPs, although the majority of methods and findings discussed will apply similarly in other cases. SNPs are given numbers by which they can be uniquely referenced. Reference numbers begin 'rs' (standing for 'reference SNP'), such as rs1205.

2.3.2 Using a genetic variant as an instrumental variable

The use of any particular genetic variant as an IV requires caution as the IV assumptions cannot be fully tested and may be violated for various epidemiological and biological reasons (see Chapter 3). As a plausible example of a valid genetic IV, in the Japanese population, a common genetic mutation in the *ALDH2* gene affects the processing of alcohol, causing excess production of a carcinogenic by-product, acetaldehyde, as well as nausea and headaches. We can use this genetic variant as an IV to assess the causal relationship between alcohol consumption and oesophageal cancer. Here, alcohol consumption is the exposure and oesophageal cancer the outcome.

Assessment of the causal relationship using classical epidemiological studies is hindered by the strong association between alcohol and tobacco smoking, another risk factor for oesophageal cancer [Davey Smith and Ebrahim, 2004]. Individuals with two copies of the *ALDH2* polymorphism tend to avoid alcohol, due to the severity of the short-term symptoms. Their risk of developing oesophageal cancer is one-third of the risk of those with no copies of the mutation [Lewis and Davey Smith, 2005]. Carriers of a single copy of this mutation exhibit only a mild intolerance to alcohol. They are still able to drink, but they cannot process the alcohol efficiently and have an increased exposure to acetaldehyde. Carriers of a single mutated allele are at three times the risk of developing oesophageal cancer compared to those without the mutation, with up to 12 times the risk in studies of heavy drinkers. The conclusion is that alcohol consumption is a cause of oesophageal cancer, since there is no association between this genetic variant and many other risk factors, and any single risk factor would have to have a massive effect on oesophageal cancer risk as well as a strong association with the genetic variant to provide an alternative explanation for these results.

These associations are summarized in Table 2.3. The genetic mutation provides a fair test to compare three populations who differ systematically only in their consumption of alcohol and exposure to acetaldehyde, and who have vastly differing risks of the outcome. The evidence for a causal link between alcohol consumption, exposure to acetaldehyde, and oesophageal cancer is compelling [Schatzkin et al., 2009]. However, in other cases, particularly if the genetic variant(s) do not explain much of the variation in the exposure, the power to detect a causal effect using a single genetic variant may be insufficient to provide such a convincing conclusion.

2.4   Classification of Mendelian randomization investigations

Not all Mendelian randomization investigations are identical in terms of how they are performed or the strength of evidence they provide. Some use a small number of genetic variants (even sometimes a single genetic variant) that have a strong and specific biological link to the exposure. Others assess the causal role of a complex exposure using a large number of genetic variants.

Genetic subgroup	Effect on alcohol metabolism	Genetic association with oesophageal cancer
Major homozygotes	No effect – can metabolize alcohol	(Reference group)
Heterozygotes	Mild effect – individuals can drink, but alcohol stays in bloodstream for longer	Increased disease risk
Minor homozygotes	Severe effect – cannot metabolize alcohol, individuals tend to abstain from alcohol	Decreased disease risk

TABLE 2.3

Example: alcohol intake and the *ALDH2* polymorphism in the Japanese population.

Sometimes, even if an exposure has a large number of genetic predictors, investigators may use a subset of those variants to assess the causal role of a particular mechanism for intervening on the exposure.

Two important categorizations relate to how many datasets are included in the analysis, and whether the analysis is performed using individual-level data or summarized data. Mendelian randomization investigations can be performed using data from a single sample (known as one-sample Mendelian randomization), in which genetic variants, exposure, and outcome are measured in the same individuals. Alternatively, in two-sample Mendelian randomization, the variant–exposure associations are estimated in one dataset and the variant–outcome associations are estimated in a second dataset [Burgess et al., 2015c]. Two-sample investigations often occur when genetic associations with the exposure are estimated in a cross-sectional sample of healthy individuals, to reflect genetic associations with usual levels of the exposure in the population, and genetic associations with a binary disease outcome are estimated in a case-control study.

A related issue is whether the analysis is performed using individual-level data or summarized data. Summarized data are genetic association estimates from regression of the exposure or outcome on a genetic variant [Burgess et al., 2013]. Several large consortia have made such estimates publicly available for hundreds of thousands of variants. Although the use of summarized data is often synonymous with the two-sample setting, the benefits and limitations for the analysis of the two choices (one- vs two-sample and individual-level vs summarized data) are distinct.

Recommendations as to how to perform a Mendelian randomization investigation are provided in Chapter 10, after we have introduced the various tools for performing an analysis and discussed their application in various examples.

2.5   Summary

Mendelian randomization has the potential to be a useful tool in a range
of scientific contexts to investigate claims of causal relationships. It must be
applied with care, as its causal claims come at the price of assumptions which
are not empirically testable. Its methods must be refined, as often data on
multiple genetic variants or data taken from several study populations are
required to achieve meaningful findings. But, when properly used, it gives
insights into the underlying causal relationships between variables which are
difficult to obtain reliably from other approaches.

3

Assumptions for causal inference

In the previous chapters, we repeatedly used the word 'causal' to describe the estimates and inferences obtained from Mendelian randomization. In this chapter, we clarify what is meant by the causal effect of an exposure on an outcome. We give a more detailed explanation of the theory of instrumental variables, and explain in biological terms various situations that may lead to violations of the instrumental variable assumptions and thus misleading causal inferences. We conclude by discussing the difference between testing for the presence of a causal relationship and estimating a causal effect, and the additional assumptions necessary for causal effect estimation.

3.1 Observational and causal relationships

As the saying goes, 'association is not causation' or in its more widely quoted form 'correlation does not imply causation'. Naive interpretation of an observed association between two variables as implying a causal relationship is a well-known logical fallacy. However, precise definitions of causality which correspond to our intuitive understanding have eluded philosophers for centuries [Pearl, 2000a]. Definitions are also complicated by the fact that, in many epidemiological contexts, causation is probabilistic rather than deterministic: for example, smoking does not always lead to lung cancer.

3.1.1 Causation as the result of manipulation

The fundamental concept in thinking about causal relationships is the idea of intervention on, or manipulation of, a variable. This is often cited as 'no causation without manipulation', reflecting that direct experimentation is necessary to demonstrate a causal effect [Holland, 1986]. A causal effect is present if the outcome differs when the exposure is set to two different levels. This differs from an observational association, which represents the difference in the outcome when the exposure is observed at two different levels. If there are variables which are correlated with the exposure, the observational association reflects differences not only in the exposure of interest, but also in variables correlated with the exposure. For the causal effect, setting the value of the exposure only alters the exposure and variables on causal pathways downstream of the exposure, not variables on alternative causal pathways.

The outcome variable Y for different observed values x of the exposure X is written as $Y|X = x$, read as Y conditional on X equalling x. Causal effects cannot be expressed in terms of observed probability distributions and so additional notation is required [Pearl, 2010]. The outcome variable Y when the exposure X is set to a given value x is written as $Y|do(X = x)$, where the *do* operator indicates that the variable is manipulated to be set to the given value.

3.1.2   Causation as a counterfactual contrast

One common definition of a causal effect is that of a counterfactual contrast [Maldonado and Greenland, 2002]. Counterfactual, literally meaning counter or contrary to fact, refers to a potential situation which could have happened, but did not [Greenland, 2000b]. For example, in the morning, Adam has a headache. He may or may not take an aspirin tablet. At the point of decision, we can conceive that there are two potential universes where Adam makes different choices about whether to take the aspirin or not. Associated with each universe is a potential outcome – does he still have a headache that afternoon? Once he has made this decision, one of these universes and outcomes becomes counterfactual; both outcomes cannot be observed. A causal effect is present if the two outcomes are different; if he still had a headache in the universe where he did not take the aspirin, but did not have a headache in the universe where he did take the aspirin, then the aspirin has caused the alleviation of the headache. With a probabilistic interpretation, assuming that the outcome is stochastic rather than deterministic, if the probability that he would still have a headache is lower in the aspirin universe than in the no-aspirin universe, then taking aspirin has a causal effect on alleviating the headache.

There are several conceptual difficulties with the counterfactual approach [Dawid, 2000]. The main difficulty is that the causal effect of an exposure for an individual can never be measured, as at least one of the two outcomes in the causal contrast is unobserved. This is referred to as the 'fundamental problem of causal inference' [Holland, 1986]. It means that a counterfactual causal estimate is not the answer to any real experiment that could be conducted, but the answer to a hypothetical experiment requiring two parallel universes. However, the counterfactual approach has many appealing features. Chiefly, it gives a precise framework for defining causal effects, aiding both informal and mathematical thinking about causal relationships.

In terms of notation, the potential outcomes that the outcome variable can take are written as $Y(x)$. If the exposure is binary, the two potential outcomes for an individual are $Y(1)$ and $Y(0)$, and the causal effect of increasing X from $X = 0$ to $X = 1$ is $Y(1) - Y(0)$.

There is some debate as to whether potential outcomes $Y(x)$ and outcomes under manipulation $Y|do(X = x)$ differ or not, but any difference is largely philosophical. In this book, we will regard these as two modes of thinking about the same concept.

3.1.3 Causation using graphical models

Graphical models, and in particular directed acyclic graphs, provide a helpful way of thinking about and expressing causal relationships. A graphical model comprises a set of nodes representing variables, and arrows representing causal effects. An arrow from variable A to variable B indicates that there is a causal effect of A on B. A graphical model need not contain all intermediate variables (such as C if $A \to C \to B$), but must contain all common causes of variables included in the graph (such as D if $A \leftarrow D \to B$). Relations between variables are expressed by directed arrows, indicating a direct causal effect, or without an arrow, indicating no direct effect. A direct causal effect is only 'direct' with respect to the variables included in the graph and as such is not direct in an absolute sense, but could act via an intermediate variable. A directed acyclic graph (DAG) is a graph that does not contain any complete cycles, such as $A \leftrightarrow B$ or $A \to B \to C \to A$; a cycle would imply that a variable is its own cause.

As an example, Figure 3.1 shows the instrumental variable (IV) assumptions (Section 2.1.2) in the form of a graph. To simplify the graph, all confounding variables are subsumed into a single 'confounder', which has effects on both the exposure and outcome. We see that there are arrows from the IV to the exposure (assumption i.), from the exposure to the outcome, and from the confounder to the exposure and to the outcome. Just as importantly, there is independence between the IV and the confounder (assumption ii.), and there is no pathway from the IV to the outcome apart from that passing through the exposure (assumption iii.), indicating that a hypothetical intervention to change the value of the IV without varying the exposure or the confounder would not affect the outcome.

3.1.4 Causation based on multivariable adjustment

Multivariable adjustment is often undertaken in the analysis of classical observational data in order to try to account for confounding. A set of covariates which, if known and conditioned on, would give an estimate of association equal to the causal effect, is referred to as 'sufficient'. Having a sufficient set of covariates is necessary to interpret the result of a multivariable-adjusted regression analysis as a causal effect. On conditioning for a sufficient set of covariates, the counterfactual outcomes at different values of the exposure should be independent of the exposure, a property known as conditional exchangeability [Greenland and Robins, 1986].

If the causal relationships between all the variables in a model representing the generating mechanism for observational data were known, a set of

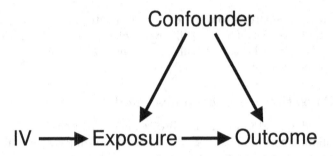

FIGURE 3.1
Directed acyclic graph illustrating instrumental variable (IV) assumptions.

covariates can be assessed as sufficient or otherwise using the 'back-door criterion' [Pearl, 2000b]. For simple causal networks, a set of covariates is sufficient if it includes all common causes of the exposure and the outcome and does not include variables on the causal pathway from the exposure to the outcome, nor common effects of the exposure and outcome. In practice, neither the underlying network of associations between variables nor the sets of all common causes and all common effects of exposure and outcome are known, and so the use of multivariable-adjusted regression analyses to assess causal effects is unreliable. It is not possible to know if adjustment for a sufficient set of covariates has been made, or if there is residual confounding due to unmeasured covariates, or if the set of covariates includes variables on the causal pathway between the exposure and outcome, whose inclusion in a regression model also biases regression coefficients. Similar arguments can be made about inverse-probability weighting and other statistical methods that exploit the back-door criterion to obtain causal estimates. This highlights the need to consider approaches for assessing causal relationships that do not make an assumption of no unmeasured confounding.

3.2   Finding a valid instrumental variable

Instrumental variable (IV) techniques represent one of the few ways available for estimating causal effects without complete knowledge of all confounders of the exposure–outcome association. We continue by recalling the properties of an IV, and discuss how the IV assumptions may be violated in practice.

3.2.1 Instrumental variable assumptions

In order for a genetic variant to be used to estimate a causal effect, it must satisfy the assumptions of an instrumental variable (Section 2.1.2), which we repeat here:

i. the variant is associated with the exposure,

ii. the variant is not associated with the outcome via a confounding pathway,

iii. the variant does not affect the outcome directly, only possibly indirectly via the exposure.

These conditions can be understood intuitively. The first assumption guarantees that genetic subgroups defined by the variant will have different average levels of the exposure. This ensures that there is a systematic difference between the subgroups. If the genetic variant is not strongly associated with the exposure (in the sense of its statistical strength of association), then it is referred to as a weak instrument (see Section 8.1). A weak instrument differs from an invalid instrument in that a weak instrument can be made stronger by collecting more data. If a single genetic variant is a weak instrument, then it will still give a valid test of the null hypothesis of no causal effect, but the power to detect a true causal effect may be low.

The second assumption can be understood as ensuring that the comparison between the genetic subgroups is a fair test, meaning that all variables other than the exposure (and downstream consequences of the exposure) are distributed equally between the subgroups. A more formal statement of the second assumption is that there is no open back-door path from the genetic variant to the outcome. This would be violated if the genetic variant were associated with a confounder of the exposure–outcome association. It would also be violated if there is a common cause of the genetic variant and the outcome, such as ancestry, unless this is adjusted for in the analysis.

The third assumption is sometimes expressed using the concept of conditional independence as 'the genetic variant is not associated with the outcome conditional on the value of the exposure and confounders of the exposure–outcome association' [Greenland, 2000a]. However, this obscures the key difference between the second and third assumptions: the second assumption relates to how the IV is distributed (it is an assumption about the associations of the IV), whereas the third assumption relates to causal pathways. The third assumption ensures that the only causal pathway (or pathways) from the genetic variant to the outcome are via the exposure. This means that the genetic variant does not directly influence the outcome, nor is there any alternative pathway by which the variant influences the outcome other than that through the exposure.

3.2.2   Validity of the IV assumptions

The counterfactual framework for causation helps understanding of when and why a randomized controlled trial (RCT) can estimate a causal effect – thought of in a counterfactual sense as a contrast between parallel universes. The randomized subgroups in an RCT can be regarded as exchangeable. This means that the same distribution of outcomes would be expected if both of the subgroups were exposed to the treatment regime (or both to the control regime). In contrast, in a typical observational analysis, the subgroups of the population with different levels of the exposure would not be exchangeable, as they differ with respect to other factors. Although an individual can only be exposed to one of the two treatment regimes (and so only observed in one universe), by exposing each subgroup to a different treatment regime, in effect we observe versions of the population in each of the two counterfactual parallel universes, and the average outcomes in each of the universes (subgroups) can be compared [Greenland and Robins, 1986]. A causal effect can be consistently estimated which represents the average effect of being assigned to the treatment group as opposed to the control group. This means that an RCT can estimate an average causal effect for the population as the contrast between the average levels of the outcome in the randomized subgroups of the population (which will have the same characteristics on average as the overall population due to the random assignment into subgroups). An individual causal effect cannot be estimated, as an individual cannot in general be subjected to both the treatment and control regimes [Rubin, 1974].

For Mendelian randomization, the similar key property of an IV is that the division of the population into genetic subgroups is independent of competing risk factors, and so genetic subgroups defined by the IV are exchangeable. For a genetic variant that divides the population into two subgroups, it is necessary that the same distribution of outcomes would have been observed in both subgroups if all individuals in both subgroups were born without the genetic variant (and the same if all individuals were born with the genetic variant). However, empirical testing of the exchangeability criterion is not possible.

We return to the question of assessing the validity of genetic variants as IVs later in this section; firstly we consider reasons why a genetic variant may not be a valid IV. These include issues of biological mechanism, genetic co-inheritance, and population effects. Invalid IVs lead to unreliable inferences for the causal effect of an exposure. The situations discussed here represent potential lack of internal validity of estimates; the question of the external validity of an IV estimate as representing the predicted effect of a clinical intervention is discussed in Chapter 6.

3.2.3 Violations of IV assumptions: Biological mechanisms

The first category of ways that we consider by which the IV assumptions may be violated is because of an underlying biological mechanism.

Pleiotropy: Pleiotropy refers to a genetic variant being associated with multiple risk factors on different causal pathways. If a genetic variant used as an IV is additionally associated with another risk factor for the outcome, then either the second or the third IV assumption is violated, and the variant is not a valid IV. If pleiotropy leads to the genetic variant being associated with the outcome via a confounding variable, then the second assumption would be violated. If pleiotropy leads to an alternative causal pathway from the variant to the outcome not via the exposure of interest, then the third assumption would be violated.

If the genetic variant is associated with an additional variable solely due to its association with the exposure of interest (called mediation or vertical pleiotropy), then this is not regarded as pleiotropy for our purposes (Figure 3.2). For example, variants in the *FTO* gene are associated with satiety (how full of food a person feels) [Wardle et al., 2008]. If satiety affects body mass index (BMI), then a variant in the *FTO* gene can be used as an IV for BMI if the two variables are on the same causal pathway, and if there is no alternative causal pathway from the genetic variant to the outcome not via BMI. However, if the *FTO* gene was also associated with (say) blood pressure, and this association was not completely mediated by the association of the gene with BMI, then it would be misleading to use a variant in the *FTO* gene to make specific inferences about the causal effect of BMI on an outcome. Figure 3.3 illustrates various scenarios by which a genetic variant may be associated with a variable other than the exposure, and discusses in each case whether the IV assumptions are valid or not.

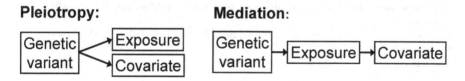

FIGURE 3.2
Illustration of the difference between pleiotropy (left, the association of the genetic variant with the covariate is independent of the exposure; sometimes called horizontal pleiotropy) and mediation (right, the association of the genetic variant with the covariate is mediated entirely via the exposure; sometimes called vertical pleiotropy).

Concerns about pleiotropy can be alleviated by using genetic variants located in genes for which the biological function is well-understood.

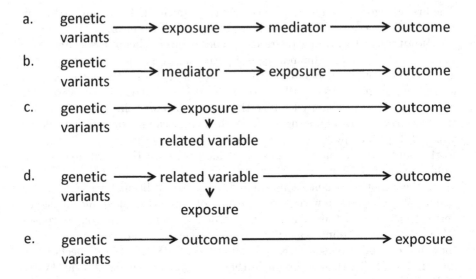

FIGURE 3.3

Diagrams illustrating validity and invalidity of instrumental variable assumptions in different scenarios.

Scenarios:

a) Mediator is on causal pathway from exposure to outcome.

b) Mediator is on causal pathway from genetic variants to exposure.

c) Genetic variants influence exposure, which has downstream effect on a related variable which does not affect the outcome.

d) Genetic variants influence a related variable, and the related variable also affects the exposure of interest.

e) Genetic variants influence the outcome primarily, and only influence the exposure via the outcome.

The related variable may be known or unknown.

In scenarios a, b, and c, as there is no alternative pathway from the genetic variants to the outcome, the instrumental variable assumptions are satisfied despite the genetic variant being associated with the mediator. In scenario d, the pathway from the genetic variants to the outcome does not pass via the exposure, and so the instrumental variable assumptions are not satisfied for the exposure (although they are satisfied for the related variable). Scenarios a, b, and c are examples of 'vertical pleiotropy' that do not invalidate the instrumental variable assumptions. Scenario d reflects a situation where the causal risk factor has been incorrectly identified – it is not the exposure, but the related variable. Scenario e reflects reverse causation, where the genetic variant has been incorrectly identified as primarily affecting the exposure; in reality, it primarily affects the outcome, and the instrumental variable assumptions are invalid.

For example, for C-reactive protein (CRP), we can use genetic variants in the *CRP* gene which are known to have functional relevance to CRP. Associations of a variant with measured covariates can be assessed to investigate potential pleiotropy, although such associations may also reflect mediation, particularly if the associations are consistent across independent variants.

Canalization: Canalization, or developmental compensation, is the phenomenon by which an individual adapts in response to genetic change in such a way that the expected effect of the change is reduced or absent [Debat and David, 2001]. It is most evident in knockout experiments, where a gene is rendered completely inactive in an organism, such as a mouse. Often the organism develops a compensatory mechanism to allow for the missing gene such that the functionality of the gene is expressed via a different biological pathway. This buffering of the genetic effect may have downstream effects on other variables. Canalization may be a problem in Mendelian randomization if groups with different levels of the genetic variants differ with respect not only to the exposure of interest, but also to other risk factors via a canalization mechanism.

In a sense, canalization is not a violation of the IV assumptions, but merely an (often unwanted) consequence. Canalization is the same process as that assessed by Mendelian randomization, as any change in other risk factors from canalization occurs as a causal effect of the genetic variant. However, the aim of Mendelian randomization is not simply to describe the effects of genetic change, but to assess the causal effect of the (non-genetic) exposure. If there is substantial canalization, Mendelian randomization estimates may be unrepresentative of clinical interventions on the exposure performed in a mature cohort.

3.2.4 Violations of IV assumptions: non-Mendelian inheritance

The second category of ways that we consider by which the IV assumptions may be violated is because of non-Mendelian inheritance. Although Mendelian principles state that genes representing separate characteristics are inherited separately, this is not always true in practice. Non-Mendelian inheritance refers to patterns of inheritance which do not correspond to Mendel's laws, specifically the law of independent assortment.

Linkage disequilibrium: One particular reason for genetic variants to be inherited together is the physical proximity of the variants on the same chromosome. Variants whose distributions are correlated are said to be in linkage disequilibrium (LD). The opposite of LD is linkage equilibrium.

LD has both desirable and undesirable consequences. If all genetic variants were truly independently distributed, then only the genetic variant which was causally responsible for variation in the exposure could be used as an IV, as other genetic variants would not be associated with the exposure. In reality, it is not necessary for the genetic variant used as the IV to be the causal variant, merely to be correlated with the causal variant [Hernán and Robins, 2006]. This is because an IV must simply divide the population into subgroups which differ systematically only with respect to the exposure. This is illustrated in Figure 3.4.

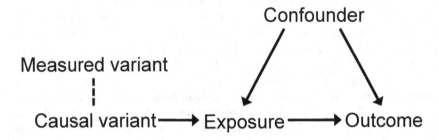

FIGURE 3.4

Diagram of instrumental variable assumptions where a variant in linkage disequilibrium with the causal variant has been measured. Such a variant would still be a valid instrumental variable. The dashed line connecting the genetic variants indicates correlation without a causal interpretation.

An undesirable consequence of LD is that genetic variants correlated with the variant used in the analysis may have effects on competing risk factors. This would lead to the violation of the second or the third IV assumption (similar to violations due to pleiotropy). Concerns about invalid inferences due to LD can be alleviated by empirical testing of the association of known potential confounders with the measured variant.

Effect modification: Effect modification is a separate phenomenon from confounding, and relates to a statistical interaction between the effect of a variable (usually an effect of the exposure) and the value of a covariate, leading to the causal effect of the exposure varying across strata defined by the covariate. Factors that may lead to effect modification include (but are not limited to) issues of non-Mendelian inheritance, such epigenetic variation [Ogbuanu et al., 2009] and parent-of-origin effects [Bochud et al., 2008].

Effect modification alone is unlikely to represent a violation of the IV assumptions. It can lead to both difficulties in interpreting Mendelian randomization investigations, but also opportunities. In the example from Section 2.3.2 of the effect of alcohol intake on oesophageal cancer risk, only men in the Japanese population tend to drink alcohol. Hence, genetic associations with the outcome may be observed only in men and may not be present in women. If there are biological reasons for genetic associations to be stronger or weaker (or even absent) in some strata of the population, then associations measured in that stratum of the population would not be representative of the effect in the population as a whole. However, this may also provide an opportunity for verifying the IV assumptions; Japanese women are a natural control group for Japanese men. If the same genetic associations of alcohol-related variants with oesophageal cancer risk seen in Japanese men are not observed in Japanese women, this provides further evidence that the genetic associations with disease risk are driven by alcohol consumption, and not by violations of the IV assumptions.

3.2.5   Violations of IV assumptions: Population effects

The final category of ways that we consider by which the IV assumptions may be violated is because of population effects.

Population stratification: Population stratification occurs when the population under investigation can be divided into distinct subpopulations. This may occur, for example, when the population is a mixture of individuals of different ethnic origins. If the frequency of the genetic variant and the distribution of the exposure are different in the different subpopulations, a spurious association between the variant and the exposure will be induced which is due to subpopulation differences, not the effect of the genetic variant. Violations of the IV assumptions may also occur if there is continuous variation in the structure of the population rather than distinct subpopulations.

Concerns about population stratification can be alleviated by restricting the study population to those with the same ethnic background (although there may still may be differences associated with ancestry in broadly-defined ethnic groups). If genetic associations are estimated in a genome-wide association study (GWAS), genomic control approaches, such as adjustment for genetic principal components, are possible. However, the use of Mendelian randomization in a population with a large amount of genetic heterogeneity is not advised.

Ascertainment effects: If the genetic variant is associated with recruitment into the study, then the relative proportions of individuals in each genetic subgroup are not the same as those in the population, and so a genetic association with the outcome in the sample may not be present in the original population. If the study cohort is a representative sample taken from the general population, ascertainment effects are unlikely to be a major problem in practice. However, if, for example, the study cohort is pregnant mothers, and the genetic variant is associated with fertility, then the distributions of the covariates in the genetic subgroups will differ and not be the same as those in the general population. This may introduce bias in the estimation of causal effects, as there is a pathway opened up from the genetic variant to the outcome by conditioning on a common cause of the variant and the outcome (referred to as collider bias, see Section 8.5).

This would also be a problem in studies looking at genetic associations in populations of diseased individuals. Individuals with greater genetically-predicted disease risk are less likely to survive to study recruitment, and so the randomization of individuals into genetic subgroups at conception at the population level would not hold in the study sample, leading to biased genetic associations in the sample.

3.2.6   Statistical assessment of the IV assumptions

Although it is not possible to demonstrate conclusively the validity of the IV assumptions, several tests and assessments are possible to increase or decrease confidence in the use of genetic variants as IVs.

The simplest assessment of instrument validity is to test the association between the genetic variant and known confounders. Association of the variant with a covariate associated with the outcome which is not on the causal pathway between the exposure and outcome would violate the second IV assumption. However, there is no definitive way to tell whether the association with the covariate is due to violation of the IV assumptions (such as by pleiotropy or linkage disequilibrium), or due to mediation through the exposure of interest. Additionally, there is no way of testing whether or not the variant is associated with an unmeasured confounder. If there are multiple covariates and/or genetic variants, then any hypothesis testing approach needs to account for the multiple comparisons of each covariate, leading to a lack of power to detect any specific association. Additionally, as several covariates may be correlated, a simple Bonferroni correction may be an over-correction. A sensible way to proceed is to combine a hypothesis testing approach with a quantitative and qualitative assessment of the imbalance of the covariates between genetic subgroups and the degree to which this may bias the IV estimate.

A further approach for testing instrument validity is to see whether the association of a genetic variant with the outcome attenuates on adjustment for the exposure [Glymour et al., 2012]. Although attenuation may not be complete even when the instrumental variable assumptions are satisfied for the exposure due to confounding and measurement error [Didelez and Sheehan, 2007], if the attenuation is not substantial then the exposure is unlikely to be on the causal pathway from the variant to the outcome.

If multiple genetic variants are available, each of which is a valid IV, then a separate IV estimate can be calculated using each of the instruments in turn. Assuming that each variant affects the exposure in a similar way, even if the genetic associations with the exposure are of different magnitude, the separate IV estimates should be similar, as they are targeting the same quantity. This can be assessed graphically by plotting the genetic associations with the exposure and outcome for each variant: a straight line through the origin is expected, as in Figure 6.1. Formally, differences between estimates can be assessed using a heterogeneity test (Section 5.3). Excess heterogeneity may be due to one or more of the variants being invalid IVs. However, the power of such tests may be limited in practice, and so testing should not be relied on for justification of the IV assumptions.

Ideally, biological knowledge rather than statistical testing should form the backbone of any justification of the use of a particular genetic variant as an IV in Mendelian randomization. The Bradford Hill guidelines form a systematic summary of common-sense principles for assessing causality in epidemiological investigations [Hill, 1965]. In Table 3.1, we apply relevant Bradford Hill guidelines for causation to Mendelian randomization as a checklist to judge whether the validity of genetic variant(s) as an IV is plausible.

3.2.7 Summary of issues relating to IV validity

The validity of IVs is of vital importance to Mendelian randomization. It is our view that the choice of genetic variants as IVs should be justified where possible by biological knowledge, although it should also be assessed by empirical statistical testing. Appropriate caution should be attached to the interpretation of Mendelian randomization findings depending on the plausibility of the IV assumptions, and particularly to those where the justification of the IV assumptions is mainly empirical. This suggests that analyses where the function of the genetic variant(s) is well-understood will be more credible than those using variants outside of gene coding regions, such as those discovered in genome-wide association studies. However, it should be remembered that all statistical methods for assessing causal effects rely on untestable assumptions, and as such, Mendelian randomization has an important role in building up the case for the causal role of a given exposure even if the validity of the IV assumptions can be challenged.

On a more positive note, a British study into the distribution of genetic variants and non-genetic factors (such as environmental exposures) in a group of blood donors and a representative sample from the population showed marked differences in the non-genetic factors, but no more difference than would be expected by chance in the genetic factors [Ebrahim and Davey Smith, 2008], indicating that genetic factors seem to be distributed independently of possible confounders in the population of the United Kingdom. This gives plausibility to the general suitability of genetic variants as IVs. However, in each specific case, the plausibility of the assumptions for the genetic variants in question should be assessed.

3.2.8 Definition of an IV as a random variable

For the more mathematically inclined, we give a further characterization of an IV in terms of random variables. We assume that we have an outcome Y that is a function of a measured exposure X and an unmeasured confounder U; that the confounding factors can be summarized by a single random variable U [Palmer et al., 2008], which satisfies the requirements of a sufficient covariate (Section 3.1.4); and that the exposure X can be expressed as a function of the confounder U and the genetic variant G. G may be a single genetic variant or a matrix corresponding to several genetic variants. The IV assumptions of Section 3.2.1 are rewritten here in terms of random variables:

- **Strength:** If a genetic association with the outcome is slight, then the association could be explained by only a small imbalance in a covariate associated with the genetic variant. Moreover, a small violation of the instrumental variable assumptions is less likely to be detected by testing the association of the variant with known covariates.
- **Consistency:** A causal relationship is more plausible if multiple independent genetic variants associated with the same exposure are all concordantly associated with the outcome, especially if the variants are located in different gene regions and/or have different mechanisms by which they influence the exposure.
- **Biological gradient:** Further, a causal relationship is more plausible if the genetic associations with the outcome and with the exposure for different variants are proportional (for example, as in Figure 6.1).
- **Specificity:** A causal relationship is more plausible if the genetic variant(s) are associated with a specific exposure and outcome, and do not have associations with a wide range of covariates and outcomes. A specific association is more likely if the genetic variant(s) are biologically proximal to the exposure, and not biologically distant. This is most likely for risk factors that are proteins or other gene products (such as C-reactive protein and fibrinogen, or gene expression), rather than more complex risk factors (such as body mass index and blood pressure).
- **Plausibility:** If the function of the genetic variant(s) is known, a causal relationship is more plausible if the mechanism by which the variant acts is credibly and specifically related to the exposure.
- **Coherence:** If an intervention on the exposure has been performed (for example, if a drug has been developed that acts on the exposure), associations with intermediate outcomes (covariates) observed in the experimental context should also be present in the genetic context; directionally concordant genetic associations should be observed with the same covariates. For example, associations of genetic variants in the *IL6R* gene region with C-reactive protein and fibrinogen should be similar to those observed for tocilizumab, an interleukin-6 receptor inhibitor [Swerdlow et al., 2012].

TABLE 3.1
Bradford Hill guidelines applied to Mendelian randomization for judging the biological plausibility of a genetic variant as an instrumental variable.

  i. G is not independent of X $(G \not\perp X)$,

 ii. G is independent of U $(G \perp U)$,

iii. G is independent of Y conditional on X and U $(G \perp Y|X,U)$.

This implies that the joint distribution of Y, X, U, G factorizes as

$$p(y, x, u, g) = p(y|u, x)p(x|u, g)p(u)p(g) \qquad (3.1)$$

which corresponds to the directed acyclic graph (DAG) in Figure 3.5 [Dawid, 2002; Didelez and Sheehan, 2007].

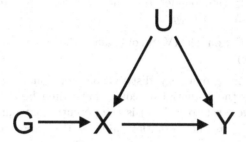

FIGURE 3.5
Directed acyclic graph of Mendelian randomization assumptions as random variables.

It is a common mistake to think that the third IV assumption should read not $G \perp Y|X,U$, but $G \perp Y|X$, implying that conditioning on U is not necessary. As X is a common descendent of G and U, conditioning on X induces an association between G and U, and therefore between G and Y. For example, if X and U are positively correlated and both have positive causal effects on Y, then conditional on X taking a value around the middle of its distribution, a large value of Y is associated with a low value of G. This is because the large value of Y is associated with a large value of U, and so G is more likely to be low and the value of X moderate and not large. The lack of independence $(G \not\perp Y|X)$ means that, in the regression of Y on X and G, the coefficient for G will generally be close to, but not equal to zero in a large sample (and especially if X is measured with error).

In order to interpret the unconfounded estimates produced by IV analysis as causal estimates, we require the additional structural assumption:

$$p(y, u, g, x|do(X = x_0)) = p(y|u, x_0)1(X = x_0)p(u)p(g) \qquad (3.2)$$

where $1(.)$ is the indicator function. This assumption links the observed distribution of Y at different values of X to the distribution of Y when setting the value of X [Didelez et al., 2010]. It relates to the consistency assumption for potential outcomes stated below.

3.2.9   Definition of an IV in potential outcomes

In the potential outcomes causal framework (Section 3.1.2), a set of outcomes $Y(x), x \in \mathfrak{X}$ are considered to exist, where $Y(x)$ is the outcome which would be observed if the exposure were set to $X = x$ and $\mathfrak{X}$ is the set of possible values of the exposure. At most one of these outcomes is ever observed. The three assumptions of Section 3.2.1 necessary for the assessment of a causal relationship can be expressed in the language of potential outcomes as follows [Angrist et al., 1996]:

i'. Relevance: $p(x|g)$ is a non-trivial function of g

ii'. Exchangeability (independence of the potential exposures and outcomes from the IV): $X(g), Y(x,g) \perp\!\!\!\perp G$.

iii'. Exclusion restriction (the IV can only affect the outcome via the exposure): $Y(x,g) = Y(x)$

where $p(x|g)$ is the probability distribution function of X conditional on $G = g$, $Y(x,g)$ is the potential outcome that would be observed if X were set to x and G were set to g, $Y(x)$ is the potential outcome observed when $X = x$, and $X(g)$ is the potential value of the exposure when $G = g$. Assumption i'. (relevance) ensures that the exposure is associated with the exposure. Assumption ii'. (exchangeability) states that the potential values of the exposure and outcome for each value of the IV are independent of the actual value of the IV. This would not be true if, for example, the IV were associated with a confounder. Assumption iii'. (exclusion restriction) states that the counterfactual values of the outcome for each value of the exposure are the same for each possible value of the IV. This means that the IV can only affect the outcome through its association with the exposure [Clarke and Windmeijer, 2012].

3.3   Testing for a causal relationship

Mendelian randomization studies are able to address two related questions: whether there is a causal effect of the exposure on the outcome, and what is the size of the causal effect [Tobin et al., 2004].

Under the assumption that the genetic variant is a valid IV, the hypothesis of a causal effect of the exposure on the outcome can be assessed by testing for independence of the variant and the outcome. A non-zero association is indicative of a causal relationship [Hernán and Robins, 2006]. The presence and direction of effect can be tested statistically by straightforward regression of the outcome on the genetic variant to see whether the estimated association is compatible with the hypothesis of no causal effect based on a chosen threshold for statistical significance.

3.3.1 Converse of the test

The converse statement to the test for a causal relationship is that if the correlation between the outcome and variant is zero, then there is no causal effect of the exposure on the outcome. Although this converse statement is not always true, as there may be zero linear correlation between the variant and outcome without independence [Spirtes et al., 2000], it is true for most biologically plausible models of the exposure–outcome association.

3.3.2 Using observational data to make causal inferences

In a natural experiment such as Mendelian randomization, as there is no intervention or manipulation of the exposure, use of the label 'causal' relies on the assumption that the observational relationships between the genetic variant(s), exposure, and outcome are informative about the structural relationship between the exposure and the outcome (structural meaning relating to the distribution of the variables under intervention). Put simply, this assumption states that the change in the outcome due to the difference in the exposure arising from the genetic variant would be the same if the exposure were intervened on to produce the same difference. This is referred to in the causal inference literature as the consistency assumption. In particular, the consistency assumption states that the outcome observed if the exposure took the value x is the same as the outcome that would have been observed if the exposure were intervened on to take the value x [VanderWeele, 2009]. Hence, although Mendelian randomization is an observational rather than an experimental technique, under this assumption it does assess a causal relationship.

3.4 Example: Lp-PLA$_2$ and coronary heart disease

To illustrate the use of Mendelian randomization to test for a causal effect, we consider the relationship between lipoprotein-associated phospholipase A$_2$ (Lp-PLA$_2$) and coronary heart disease (CHD) risk. Lp-PLA$_2$ was proposed as a potential causal risk factor for CHD based on observational studies and some experimental research. Darapladib is a drug that was developed as an inhibitor of Lp-PLA$_2$. It was shown to be successful in lowering Lp-PLA$_2$ in early-phase clinical trials, and was taken forward to large-scale Phase III trials. However, trials including 13 026 patients with a median follow-up of 2.5 years [O'Donoghue et al., 2014] and 15 828 patients with a median follow-up of 3.7 years [Stability Investigators, 2014] both failed to show efficacy in reducing the rate of major coronary events. The financial burden of these failed trials was monumental, in excess of a billion US dollars. Our question is: could genetic evidence have predicted this outcome?

We consider six different genetic variants located in the *PLA2G7* gene, the gene encoding Lp-PLA$_2$: rs76863441 (also called Val279Phe), a loss-of-function (LoF) variant with a large effect on Lp-PLA$_2$ that is relatively widespread in East Asians; rs142974898, rs144983904, rs76863441, and rs140020965, four LoF variants with large effects on Lp-PLA$_2$ that are rare, but encountered in Europeans and South Asians; and rs1051931 (Val379Ala), a variant with a modest effect but which is relatively common in Europeans. Full results were reported in Gregson et al. [2017]; we provide a summary of the headline results here.

Figure 3.6 shows the associations of the variants with Lp-PLA$_2$ activity as well as with various other cardiovascular risk factors. Also shown are the associations of darapladib from the randomized trials. We see that the genetic variants are robustly associated with Lp-PLA$_2$ activity, but not associated with a broad range of potential confounders. While this does not prove the validity of the genetic variants as IVs, it provides supportive evidence.

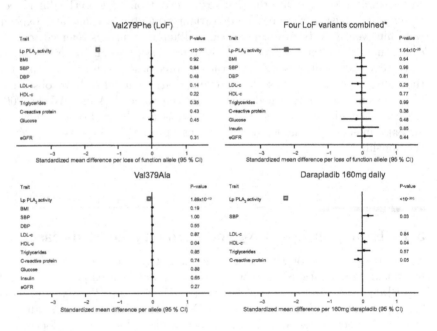

FIGURE 3.6

Mean differences in Lp-PLA$_2$ activity and cardiovascular risk factor levels per Lp-PLA$_2$-lowering allele or with darapladib taken daily. * = combined association for any of four rare loss-of-function (LoF) variants. Lines represent 95% confidence intervals. Taken from Gregson et al. [2017].

Figure 3.7 shows the associations of the variants with CHD risk. There is no evidence that any of the variants are associated with CHD risk. In each case, the 95% confidence interval for the genetic association with CHD risk overlaps the null. This shows that subgroups of the population with genetic variants that predispose individuals to having lifelong lower levels of Lp-PLA$_2$ do not differ in their risk of CHD compared to subgroups of the population who do not have these variants. The implication is that pharmacological agents that lower Lp-PLA$_2$ levels (such as darapladib) are not likely to reduce CHD risk, as was observed in the clinical trials. If this information had been available previously, then two costly trials could have been avoided, and resources could have been focused on other cardiovascular risk factors.

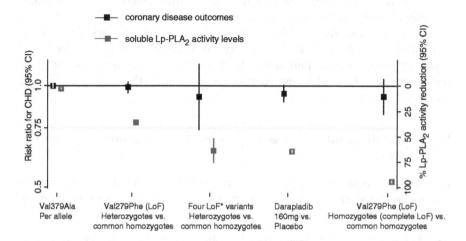

FIGURE 3.7
Association of Lp-PLA$_2$-lowering alleles with Lp-PLA$_2$ activity (grey estimates) and CHD risk (black estimates). * = combined association for any of four rare loss-of-function (LoF) variants. Lines represent 95% confidence intervals. Taken from Gregson et al. [2017].

3.5 Estimating a causal effect

Although testing for a causal relationship is useful and may be sufficient in some cases, there are several reasons why it is desirable to go beyond this and to estimate the size of a causal effect. First, this is usually the parameter representing the answer to the question of interest. Secondly, with multiple genetic variants, greater power can be achieved. If several independent IVs all have a concordant association with the outcome, the overall estimate of causal effect using all the IVs may provide evidence for a causal effect at a desired level of statistical significance even if none of the estimates from the individual IVs do. Thirdly, often a null effect is expected. By estimating a confidence interval for the causal effect, we obtain bounds on its plausible size. Although it is not statistically possible to prove the null hypothesis, it may be possible to obtain a sample size large enough such that the confidence interval bounds for the causal effect are narrow enough that the range of plausible causal effect values excludes a minimally clinically relevant causal effect. Fourthly, comparing the causal estimates from different genetic variants is a way of assessing instrument validity.

In this section, we consider technical issues associated with parameter estimation: the assumptions necessary to estimate a causal effect, and definitions of the causal parameters to be estimated. Having discussed these points, we proceed in the next chapter to consider methods for constructing different IV estimators.

3.5.1   Additional IV assumptions for estimating a causal effect

In order to estimate a causal effect, it is necessary to make further assumptions to the ones listed in Section 3.2.1 [Angrist et al., 1996]. There are two distinct assumptions that are commonly made:

- Monotonicity, which means that any change in the exposure from varying the IV should be in the same direction (an increase or a decrease) for all individuals in the population.

- Homogeneity, which means that the causal effect of the exposure on the outcome is constant for all individuals in the population.

The monotonicity assumption is credible for most biologically plausible situations in which Mendelian randomization investigations for estimating a causal effect are undertaken. In the potential outcomes notation, monotonicity implies that as the value of G increases for all individuals, the potential values of the exposure $X(g)$ are increasing for all individuals in the population, or decreasing for all individuals in the population: for a biallelic SNP, this means either $X(0) \geq X(1) \geq X(2)$ for each individual, or $X(2) \geq X(1) \geq X(0)$ for each individual. It would not be a plausible assumption in the example from Section 2.3.2 of the effect of alcohol intake on oesophageal cancer risk, as the average levels of alcohol intake and the associated disease risk are not monotone in the number of variant alleles.

If the monotonicity assumption is not plausible, then a causal effect can be identified under a homogeneity assumption. The simplest version of this assumption is that the causal effect has the same magnitude in all individuals (that is, there is no effect modification). Weaker versions of this assumption can be expressed: for example, we can assume that there is no effect modification at each level of the IV [Swanson and Hernán, 2013].

Under the monotonicity assumption, an IV estimate represents a local average treatment effect (also called a complier-average causal effect). This is the average causal effect amongst individuals whose exposure value is influenced by the IV. Such individuals are referred to as 'compliers'. This may be the whole population; an example where it is a subset of the population is for the exposure of alcohol intake, where individuals who abstain from alcohol for cultural or religious reasons would do so regardless of their IV value, and so would not be compliers. Under the homogeneity assumption, the causal effect is constant in the population, and so the IV estimate represents an average causal effect. The word 'average' allows the causal relationship to be stochastic, rather than deterministic.

When the exposure is a continuous variable (as opposed to a binary or categorical variable), common practice is to assume a linear causal relationship between the exposure and the outcome. This is partly pragmatic; otherwise, an investigator would not be able to summarize the causal effect of the exposure as a single numerical value. A practical reason is that genetic variants typically influence a risk factor by shifting its distribution. As Mendelian randomization compares the average outcome in genetic subgroups of the population comprising individuals with a range of exposure values, the genetic association with the outcome represents the impact of a population shift in the exposure distribution, rather than the causal effect of changing the exposure from one particular value to another. While it is possible to estimate how the causal effect of the exposure varies at different values of the exposure using Mendelian randomization, the estimation of non-linear causal effects requires additional assumptions as well as individual-level data on the exposure, outcome, and genetic variants in the same individuals; see Section 9.3 for details.

3.5.2 Well-defined interventions

While Mendelian randomization aims to address the question of whether a risk factor is a cause of an outcome, in reality this is not a well-defined question. For example, in considering the question 'would lowering body mass index (BMI) reduce cardiovascular mortality?', several further questions arise. How is BMI proposed to be lowered? – by increasing metabolism? by suppressing appetite? How long is BMI proposed to be lowered for? To whom will the intervention be applied? To answer the question 'is high BMI a cause of increased cardiovascular mortality?', one first has to pose the question in a precise way.

There are additional technical assumptions required for causal estimation. The 'no interference' assumption (also called the 'stable unit treatment value assumption') states that the potential outcomes for each individual should be unaffected by how the exposure was assigned, and unaffected by variables in the model relating to other individuals [Cox, 1958]. There is also the 'no multiple versions of treatment' assumption, which states that the value of the outcome is the same when the exposure is set to take a certain value independently of how the exposure was manipulated or altered to take that value. These assumptions are required by all methods for causal inference so that causal estimates can be interpreted in the way one would expect.

The 'no multiple versions of treatment' is generally not plausible, as the impact on the outcome typically varies depending on how the exposure is varied: the duration of the intervention, the timing of the intervention, the magnitude of the intervention, and the mechanism of the intervention. In particular, the change in an outcome resulting from a genetic change in the exposure may well differ from the change resulting from a pharmacological or clinical intervention on the exposure. Estimates from Mendelian randomization should therefore not be interpreted naively as the expected impact of an intervention in the exposure of interest in practice. The aim of Mendelian randomization is therefore less about estimating a specific causal effect, and more about finding evidence to support a causal hypothesis. Causal estimates are primarily useful insofar as they provide a valid test of the causal null hypothesis, which is that intervention on the exposure does not lead to changes in the outcome. We return to discuss this point in Chapter 6. However, even if these assumptions are not always plausible, it is instructive to think carefully about what causal parameters can be estimated if these assumptions are satisfied.

3.5.3   Causal parameters

The average causal effect (ACE) of an exposure [Didelez and Sheehan, 2007] is the expected difference in the outcome when the exposure is set to two different values:

$$ACE(x_0, x_1) = \quad \text{Expected outcome when the exposure is set at } x_1$$
$$- \text{expected outcome when the exposure is set at } x_0. \quad (3.3)$$

This can be written as:

$$ACE(x_0, x_1) = \mathbb{E}(Y|do(X = x_1)) - \mathbb{E}(Y|do(X = x_0)). \quad (3.4)$$

With a binary outcome ($Y = 0$ or 1), the average causal effect is also called the causal risk difference. However, it is often more natural to consider a causal risk ratio (CRR) or causal odds ratio (COR):

$$CRR(x_0, x_1) = \frac{\text{Probability of outcome when the exposure is set at } x_1}{\text{Probability of outcome when the exposure is set at } x_0},$$
(3.5)

$$COR(x_0, x_1) = \frac{\text{Odds of outcome when the exposure is set at } x_1}{\text{Odds of outcome when the exposure is set at } x_0}.$$
(3.6)

These can be written as:

$$CRR(x_0, x_1) = \frac{\mathbb{P}(Y = 1 | do(X = x_1))}{\mathbb{P}(Y = 1 | do(X = x_0))},$$
(3.7)

$$COR(x_0, x_1) = \frac{\mathbb{P}(Y = 1 | do(X = x_1))\mathbb{P}(Y = 0 | do(X = x_0))}{\mathbb{P}(Y = 1 | do(X = x_0))\mathbb{P}(Y = 0 | do(X = x_1))}.$$
(3.8)

If the exposure is binary, then the average causal effect has a single meaningful value: the average effect on the outcome at $X = 1$ versus $X = 0$. Similarly for the causal risk ratio and causal odds ratio. For a continuous exposure, under the assumption of linearity in the causal effect of the exposure on the outcome on an additive scale, the average causal effect is a constant function of the difference between x_1 and x_0, and is therefore often expressed as the average effect on the outcome per unit change in the exposure on an additive scale. Under the assumption of log-linearity (linearity on a multiplicative scale), the causal risk ratio is a constant function of the difference between x_1 and x_0, and is therefore often expressed as the average effect on the outcome on a multiplicative scale per unit change in the exposure. This is sometimes referred to as a relative risk estimate.

The linearity assumption on an additive scale is that the expected value of the outcome Y conditional on the exposure X and confounders U is:

$$\mathbb{E}(Y | X = x, U = u) = \theta_0 + \theta_1 x + h(u)$$
(3.9)

where $h(u)$ is a function of the confounding variables U, meaning that additionally there is no interaction term between X and U in the conditional expectation of Y (no effect modification by U). It is also required that the structural model:

$$\mathbb{E}(Y | do(X = x)) = \theta_0' + \theta_1 x$$
(3.10)

holds, where the causal effect θ_1 is the same as in the equation above. The parameter θ_1 represents the average causal effect for a unit change in the exposure. The log-linearity assumption is similar, except that the left-hand side of the two equations is prefixed by the logarithm function:

$$\log(\mathbb{E}(Y | X = x, U = u)) = \theta_0 + \theta_1 x + h(u)$$
(3.11)

and:

$$\log(\mathbb{E}(Y | do(X = x))) = \theta_0' + \theta_1 x$$
(3.12)

for some θ_0, θ_0', θ_1, and $h(u)$ as above. In this case, $\exp(\theta_1)$ represents the causal risk ratio for a unit change in the exposure, where exp is the exponential function.

While it is possible to consider a model that is logit-linear in the causal effect of the exposure on the outcome (where logit is the link function used in logistic regression), an interpretation of the causal odds ratio $\exp(\theta_1)$ as the odds ratio for the outcome per unit change in the exposure is not technically correct. This is due to the non-collapsibility of the odds ratio. However, this issue is usually of little practical concern, and the IV estimate expressed as a causal odds ratio does have an interpretation as the odds ratio for the outcome of a population shift in the distribution of the exposure [Burgess and CCGC, 2013]. Causal odds ratios differ depending on the distribution of the exposure and the choice of covariate adjustment in the analysis model, even if these covariates are not confounders, although differences in practice are often slight [Burgess, 2017]. We return to this issue in Section 8.7.

3.6 Summary

The instrumental variable assumptions make assessment of causation in an observational setting possible even without complete knowledge of all the confounders of the exposure–outcome association. Genetic variants have good theoretical and empirical plausibility for use as instrumental variables in general, but there are several reasons why the instrumental variable assumptions may be violated for a specific genetic variant and exposure.

We continue in the next chapter to consider methods for estimating the size of a causal effect using instrumental variables.

4

Estimating a causal effect from individual-level data

In this chapter, we discuss estimation of causal effects using instrumental variables for both continuous and binary outcomes based on individual-level data. We focus attention on the case of a single continuous exposure variable, as this is the usual situation in Mendelian randomization. The same methods can be used in the case of a single binary exposure, although there are some nuances regarding the interpretation of the estimate (Section 8.11). We here present the ratio and two-stage methods, which assume that genetic variants are all valid instrumental variables. More sophisticated methods relaxing this assumption are introduced in later chapters. We also provide code for implementing the methods using standard statistical software packages.

4.1   Ratio of coefficients method

The ratio of coefficients method, or the Wald method [Wald, 1940], is the simplest way of estimating the causal effect of the exposure (X) on the outcome (Y). The ratio method uses a single instrumental variable (IV). If more than one variant is available which is a valid IV then the causal estimates from the ratio method using each variant can be calculated separately, or the variants can be combined into a single IV in an allele score approach (Section 8.2). Alternatively, the two-stage methods described in the next section can be used.

4.1.1   Continuous outcome, dichotomous IV

We initially assume that we have an IV G which takes the values 0 or 1, dividing the population into two genetic subgroups. The IV can be thought of as a single nucleotide polymorphism (SNP) where two of the three subgroups are merged together, for example, reflecting a dominant or recessive genetic model, or because there are very few individuals in the least common genetic subgroup (the minor homozygotes). In a recessive model, a single copy of the major (wildtype) allele A is sufficient to mask a minor (variant) allele; the genetic subgroups are AA/Aa (major homozygote/heterozygote) and aa (minor homozygote). A dominant model is similar, except that the heterozygotes are combined with the minor homozygotes; the two genetic subgroups are AA and Aa/aa.

From the IV assumptions, the distribution of the exposure differs in the two genetic subgroups. If the distribution of the outcome also differs, then there is a causal effect of the exposure on the outcome. We define $\bar{Y}_j$ for $j = 0, 1$ as the average value of outcome for all individuals with genotype $G = j$, and define $\bar{X}_j$ similarly for the exposure. Figure 4.1 displays the mean exposure and outcome in the two genetic subgroups in a fictitious example with a positive causal effect of X on Y.

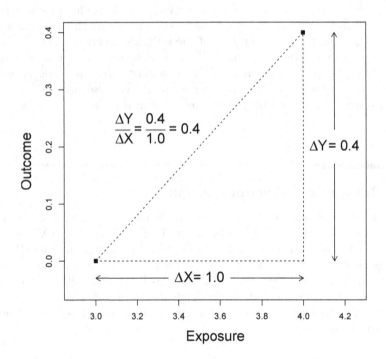

FIGURE 4.1

Points representing mean exposure and outcome in two genetic subgroups with IV ratio estimate.

We see that an average difference in the exposure between the two subgroups of $\Delta X = \bar{X}_1 - \bar{X}_0$ results in an average difference in the outcome of $\Delta Y = \bar{Y}_1 - \bar{Y}_0$. The ratio estimate for the change in outcome due to a unit increase in the exposure is:

$$\text{Ratio method estimate (dichotomous IV)} = \frac{\Delta Y}{\Delta X} = \frac{\bar{Y}_1 - \bar{Y}_0}{\bar{X}_1 - \bar{X}_0}. \qquad (4.1)$$

In the example shown (Figure 4.1), $\Delta Y = 0.4$ and $\Delta X = 1.0$, giving a ratio estimate of $\frac{0.4}{1.0} = 0.4$. Assuming that the effect of the exposure on the outcome is linear with no effect modification by confounders, this is a consistent estimate of the average causal effect as defined in Section 3.5.3 [Didelez et al., 2010]. The term 'consistent' means that the estimate tends towards the true value of the causal effect as the sample size increases, and would attain the true value in a hypothetical infinite sample. If the effect is not linear, then the ratio estimate approximates the average causal effect of a population shift in the distribution of the exposure [Burgess et al., 2014a].

IV estimates are usually expressed as the change in the outcome resulting from a unit increase in the exposure, although changes in the outcome corresponding to different magnitudes of change in the exposure could be quoted instead. For example, if the exposure is lipoprotein(a) measured in mg/dL units, then the causal estimate represents the effect of a 1 mg/dL increase in lipoprotein(a). Assuming linearity, the effect of a 10 mg/dL increase in lipoprotein(a) can be obtained by multiplying the ratio estimate by 10. The effect of a 15 mg/dL decrease in lipoprotein(a) can be obtained by multiplying the ratio estimate by -15. The IV estimate may also be expressed per standard deviation increase (or decrease) in the exposure. This is necessary if the exposure has been standardized to be normally distributed (for example, using a rank-based inverse normal transformation). If an IV estimate is expressed for a change in the exposure much greater than the association of the genetic variant with the exposure, a linear extrapolation may not be justified. However, some extrapolation may be desirable to scale the causal estimate to a clinically relevant magnitude of change in the exposure.

4.1.2 Continuous outcome, polytomous or continuous IV

Alternatively, the IV may not be dichotomous, but polytomous (takes more than two distinct values). This is the usual case for a biallelic SNP; the three levels AA (major homozygote), Aa (heterozygote), and aa (minor homozygote) will be referred to as 0, 1, and 2, corresponding to the number of minor alleles (here the minor allele is taken as the effect allele). In an additive or 'per allele' model, we assume that the association of the genetic variant with the exposure is proportional to the number of variant alleles. The IV could also be a continuous allele score (Section 8.2), under the assumption that the association of the score with the exposure is linear.

The coefficient of G in the regression of X on G is here written as $\hat{\beta}_{X|G}$, and represents the change in X for a unit change in G. Similarly, the coefficient of G in the regression of Y on G is written as $\hat{\beta}_{Y|G}$. The ratio estimate of the causal effect is:

$$\text{Ratio method estimate (polytomous/continuous IV)} = \frac{\hat{\beta}_{Y|G}}{\hat{\beta}_{X|G}}. \qquad (4.2)$$

Intuitively, we can think of the ratio method as saying that the change in Y for a unit increase in X is equal to the change in Y for a unit increase in G, scaled by the change in X for a unit increase in G. Again, this is a consistent estimate of the average causal effect under the assumption of linearity with no effect modification by confounders.

Illustrative synthetic data for an IV taking three values are shown in Figure 4.2. Each of the graphs is plotted on the same scale. The top-left panel shows that the exposure and outcome are negatively correlated, with the line showing the observational association from linear regression. However, as shown in the top-right panel, where individuals in different genetic subgroups are marked with different plotting symbols, individuals in the subgroup marked with circles tend to congregate towards the south-west of the graph and individuals in the subgroup marked with squares tend towards the north-east of the graph. The bottom-left panel shows the mean values of the exposure and outcome in each genetic subgroup with lines representing 95% confidence intervals intervals for the means. The bottom-right panel includes the individual data points, the subgroup means and the causal estimate from the ratio method. We see that the causal estimate is positive. The negative correlation within each subgroup reflects the influence of confounders, but the positive trend in the subgroup means reflects the unconfounded relationship between the exposure and outcome. The 95% confidence intervals for the lines passing through the points show that the uncertainty in the ratio IV estimate is greater than that of the observational estimate.

We note that the ratio estimate can be calculated simply from the coefficients $\hat{\beta}_{X|G}$ and $\hat{\beta}_{Y|G}$, and as such only requires the availability of summarized data, not individual-level data. Methods for obtaining IV estimates using summarized data are discussed further in Chapter 5.

4.1.3 Binary outcome

Generally in epidemiological applications, disease is the outcome of interest. Disease outcomes are often binary (that is, they are dichotomous and take values zero or one). We use the epidemiological terminology of referring to an individual with an outcome event as a case ($Y = 1$), and an individual with no event as a control ($Y = 0$).

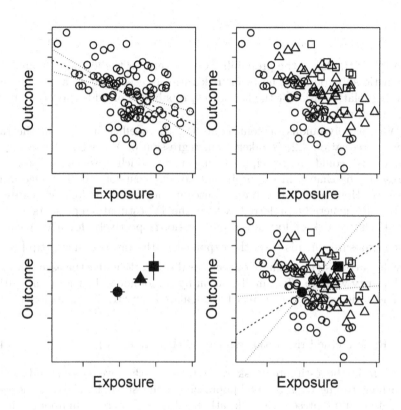

FIGURE 4.2
Illustration of ratio method for polytomous IV taking three values with a continuous outcome in a fictitious dataset: (top-left) exposure and outcome for all individuals, observational estimate with 95% confidence interval; (top-right) individuals divided into genetic subgroups by plot symbol; (bottom-left) mean exposure and outcome in each genetic subgroup (lines represent 95% confidence intervals); (bottom-right) ratio IV estimate with 95% confidence interval.

With a binary outcome and a dichotomous IV, the ratio estimate is defined similarly as with a continuous outcome:

$$\text{Ratio method log risk ratio estimate (dichotomous IV)} = \frac{\Delta Y}{\Delta X} \quad (4.3)$$

$$= \frac{\bar{Y}_1 - \bar{Y}_0}{\bar{X}_1 - \bar{X}_0}$$

where $\bar{Y}_j$ is the log of the probability of an event, or the log odds of an event, in genetic subgroup j. The term 'risk ratio' is used here as a generic term meaning relative risk (for the log of the probability) or odds ratio (for the log odds) as appropriate.

With a polytomous or continuous IV, the coefficient $\hat{\beta}_{Y|G}$ in the ratio estimate (equation 4.2) is taken from regression of Y on G. The regression model used could in principle be linear, in which case the IV estimate represents the change in the probability of an event for a unit change in the exposure. However, with a binary outcome, log-linear or logistic regression models are generally preferred, where the IV estimate represents the log causal relative risk or log causal odds ratio, respectively, for a unit change in the exposure. In this case, the exponent of the ratio estimate $\exp\left(\frac{\hat{\beta}_{Y|G}}{\hat{\beta}_{X|G}}\right)$ provides a consistent estimate of the causal risk ratio under the assumption of log-linearity with no effect modification by confounders [Didelez et al., 2010].

The ratio estimate can also be calculated directly in an exponentiated form:

$$\text{Ratio method risk ratio estimate (dichotomous IV)} = R^{1/\Delta X} \quad (4.4)$$

where R is the estimated risk ratio between the two genetic subgroups. Returning to the example of lipoprotein(a) measured in mg/dL, the ratio estimate would represent the risk ratio per 1 mg/dL increase in lipoprotein(a). To express the ratio estimate as a risk ratio for a 10 mg/dL increase in lipoprotein(a), the log risk ratio is multiplied by 10 before exponentiating.

4.1.4   Retrospective and case-control data

In Mendelian randomization, when retrospective data are available, it is usual to make inferences on the genetic associations with the exposure using only non-diseased individuals, such as the control population in a case-control study [Minelli et al., 2004]. This makes the assumption that the distribution of the exposure in the controls is similar to that of the general population, which is true for a rare disease [Bowden and Vansteelandt, 2011]. This is necessary to prevent bias of the causal estimate for two reasons. The first reason is reverse causation, whereby post-event measurements of the exposure may be distorted by the outcome event. Secondly, in a case-control setting, over-recruitment of cases into the study means that the distribution of confounders in the ascertained population is different to that in the general population. An association is then induced between the IV and the confounders, leading to possible bias in the IV estimate [Didelez and Sheehan, 2007]. This affects not only the ratio method, but all IV methods.

If the outcome is common and its prevalence in the population from which the case-control sample was taken is known, such as in a nested case-control study, then inferences on the genetic associations with the exposure can be obtained using both cases and controls, provided that measurements of the exposure in cases were taken prior to the outcome event. This analysis can be performed by weighting the sample so that the proportions of cases and controls in the reweighted sample match those in the underlying population [Bowden and Vansteelandt, 2011].

4.1.5 Confidence intervals

Confidence intervals for the ratio estimate can be calculated in several ways.

Normal approximation: The simplest way is to use a normal approximation. With a continuous outcome, standard errors (SEs) and confidence intervals from the two-stage least squares method, introduced below, are given in standard software commands (Section 4.4). Alternatively, the following approximation can be used, based on the first two terms of the delta method expansion for the variance of a ratio [Thomas et al., 2007]:

$$\text{Standard error of ratio estimate} \simeq \sqrt{\frac{\text{se}(\hat{\beta}_{Y|G})^2}{\hat{\beta}_{X|G}^2} + \frac{\hat{\beta}_{Y|G}^2 \,\text{se}(\hat{\beta}_{X|G})^2}{\hat{\beta}_{X|G}^4}} \quad (4.5)$$

where $\text{se}(\hat{\beta}_{Y|G})$ is the standard error of $\hat{\beta}_{Y|G}$ and $\text{se}(\hat{\beta}_{X|G})$ is the standard error of $\hat{\beta}_{X|G}$. This approximation assumes that the numerator and denominator of the ratio estimator are uncorrelated; such correlation could be accounted for by including a third term of the delta expansion:

$$\text{SE} \simeq \sqrt{\frac{\text{se}(\hat{\beta}_{Y|G})^2}{\hat{\beta}_{X|G}^2} + \frac{\hat{\beta}_{Y|G}^2 \,\text{se}(\hat{\beta}_{X|G})^2}{\hat{\beta}_{X|G}^4} + \frac{\hat{\beta}_{Y|G}\,\rho\,\text{se}(\hat{\beta}_{Y|G})\,\text{se}(\hat{\beta}_{X|G})}{\hat{\beta}_{X|G}^3}} \quad (4.6)$$

where ρ is the correlation between $\hat{\beta}_{Y|G}$ and $\hat{\beta}_{X|G}$ [Thomas et al., 2007]. This correlation is difficult to estimate in practice, although typically its value does not substantially affect the standard error estimate.

If the uncertainty in the genetic association with the exposure is small compared to the uncertainty in the genetic association with the outcome, then a simpler approximation can be used based on the first-order term of the delta expansion only:

$$\text{Standard error of ratio estimate} \simeq \left| \frac{\text{se}(\hat{\beta}_{Y|G})}{\hat{\beta}_{X|G}} \right| \quad (4.7)$$

where $|.|$ indicates to take the positive value of a quantity (as a standard error cannot be negative). This approximation only accounts for uncertainty in the genetic association with the outcome. We refer to equations (4.5) and (4.6) as second-order standard errors and equation (4.7) as the first-order standard error estimate.

However, for either approximation, asymptotic (large sample) normal approximations may result in overly narrow confidence intervals, especially if the sample size is not large or the IV is 'weak' (see Section 8.1). This is because IV estimates are not truly normally distributed.

Fieller's theorem: If the regression coefficients in the ratio method $\hat{\beta}_{Y|G}$ and $\hat{\beta}_{X|G}$ are assumed to be normally distributed, critical values and confidence intervals for the ratio estimator may be calculated using Fieller's theorem [Fieller, 1954; Lawlor et al., 2008]. We assume that the correlation between $\hat{\beta}_{Y|G}$ and $\hat{\beta}_{X|G}$ is zero; other values can be used, but the impact on the confidence interval is usually small [Minelli et al., 2004]. If the standard errors are $\text{se}(\hat{\beta}_{Y|G})$ and $\text{se}(\hat{\beta}_{X|G})$ and the sample size is N, then we define:

$$
\begin{aligned}
f_0 &= \hat{\beta}_{Y|G}{}^2 - t_N(0.975)^2 \, \text{se}(\hat{\beta}_{Y|G})^2 \qquad\qquad (4.8)\\
f_1 &= \hat{\beta}_{X|G}{}^2 - t_N(0.975)^2 \, \text{se}(\hat{\beta}_{X|G})^2 \\
f_2 &= \hat{\beta}_{Y|G} \, \hat{\beta}_{X|G} \\
D &= f_2{}^2 - f_0 f_1
\end{aligned}
$$

where $t_N(0.975)$ is the 97.5th percentile point of a t-distribution with N degrees of freedom (for $N > 100$, $t_N(0.975) \approx 1.96$).

If $D > 0$ and $f_1 > 0$, then the 95% confidence interval is from $(f_2 - \sqrt{D})/f_1$ to $(f_2 + \sqrt{D})/f_1$. The confidence interval is more likely to be a closed interval like this if we have a 'strong' instrument (that is, an instrument which is statistically strongly associated with the exposure). Confidence intervals of size α can be similarly constructed by using the $(1 - \alpha/2)$ point of the t-distribution.

If $D < 0$, then there is no interval which covers the true parameter with 95% confidence. This occurs when there is little differentiation in both the exposure and outcome distributions between the genetic subgroups, and so a gradient corresponding to any size of causal effect is plausible. The only valid 95% confidence interval is the unbounded interval from minus infinity to plus infinity. An example where Fieller's theorem would give an unbounded confidence interval is displayed in Figure 4.3. This situation is likely to occur when the IV explains little of the variation in the exposure; it is a weak instrument.

If $D > 0$ and $f_1 < 0$, then the 95% confidence interval is the union of two intervals from minus infinity to $(f_2 + \sqrt{D})/f_1$ and from $(f_2 - \sqrt{D})/f_1$ to plus infinity. All possible values are included in the interval except those between $(f_2 + \sqrt{D})/f_1$ and $(f_2 - \sqrt{D})/f_1$. An example where Fieller's theorem would give such a confidence interval including infinity but excluding zero,

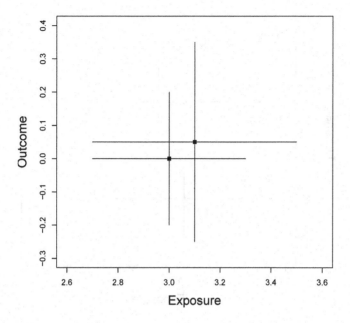

FIGURE 4.3

Points representing mean exposure and outcome (lines are 95% confidence intervals) in two genetic subgroups where the confidence interval from Fieller's theorem for the ratio estimate is unbounded.

is displayed in Figure 4.4. This suggests that the differences in the outcome are not caused solely by differences in the exposure, and so the IV assumptions appear to be violated.

To summarize, Fieller's theorem gives confidence intervals that have one of three possible forms [Buonaccorsi, 2005]:

i. The interval may be a closed interval $[a, b]$,

ii. The interval may be the complement of a closed interval $(-\infty, b] \cup [a, \infty)$,

iii. The interval may be unbounded.

Confidence intervals from Fieller's theorem are preferred to those from an asymptotic normal approximation when the IV is weak. A tool to calculate confidence intervals from Fieller's theorem based on the associations of the IV with the exposure and the outcome is available online (https://sb452.shinyapps.io/fieller/).

Alternative approaches for inference with weak instruments not discussed further here are confidence based on inverting a test statistic, such as the Anderson–Rubin test statistic [Anderson and Rubin, 1949] or the conditional likelihood ratio test statistic [Moreira, 2003]. These intervals give appropriate

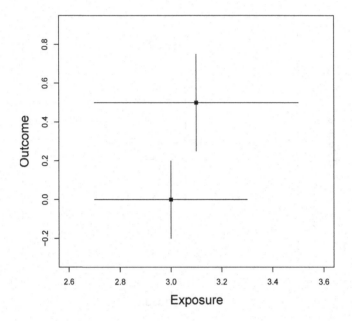

FIGURE 4.4

Points representing mean exposure and outcome (lines are 95% confidence intervals) in two genetic subgroups where the confidence interval from Fieller's theorem for the ratio estimate is compatible with infinity (vertical line), but not zero (horizontal line).

confidence levels under the null hypothesis with weak instruments, but may be underpowered with stronger instruments.

4.1.6   Reduced power of IV analyses

Figure 4.2 illustrates the wider confidence interval of an IV estimate compared with that of an observational estimate. As in many areas of applied statistics, there is a trade-off in choice of estimation procedure between bias and variance. The observational estimate is precisely estimated, but typically biased for the causal effect, whereas the IV estimate is unbiased, but typically imprecisely estimated. The loss of precision in the IV estimate is the cost of unbiased estimation. When making causal assessments, we would argue that no appreciable amount of bias should be introduced in order to reduce the variance of the estimate [Zohoori and Savitz, 1997].

However, the sample size required to obtain precise enough causal estimates to be clinically relevant can be very large [Ebrahim and Davey Smith, 2008]. A rule of thumb for power is that the sample size for a conventional analysis should be divided by the coefficient of determination

(R^2) of the IV on the exposure (Section 8.9). For example, if the sample size for an observational regression analysis of the outcome on the exposure to detect a given effect size requires a sample size of 400, and the IV explains 2% of the variation in the exposure, then the sample size required for an IV analysis is approximately $400/0.02 = 20\,000$. For this reason, while in some cases the ratio method may be sufficient for the analysis in question, we are motivated to consider methods which can incorporate data on more than one IV, and hence give more precise estimates of causal effects.

4.2 Two-stage methods

A two-stage method comprises two regression stages: the first-stage regression of the exposure on the genetic IVs, and the second-stage regression of the outcome on the fitted values of the exposure from the first stage.

4.2.1 Continuous outcome – two-stage least squares

With continuous outcomes and a linear model, the two-stage method is known as two-stage least squares (2SLS). It can be used with multiple IVs, which may be correlated or uncorrelated. In the first-stage (G–X) regression, the exposure is regressed on the IV (or IVs) to give fitted values of the exposure ($\hat{X}|G$). In the second-stage (X–Y) regression, the outcome is regressed on the fitted values for the exposure from the first stage regression. The causal estimate is this second-stage regression coefficient for the change in outcome caused by a unit change in the exposure.

With a single IV, the 2SLS estimate is the same as the ratio estimate. With multiple IVs, the 2SLS estimator may be viewed as a weighted mean of the ratio estimates calculated using the instruments one at the time, where the weights are determined by the relative strengths of the instruments in the first-stage regression [Angrist et al., 2000; Angrist and Pischke, 2009a].

Suppose we have J instrumental variables. With data on individuals indexed by $i = 1, \ldots, N$ who have exposure x_i, outcome y_i and assuming an additive per allele model for the IVs g_{ij} indexed by $j = 1, \ldots, J$, the first-stage regression model is:

$$x_i = \beta_0 + \sum_j \beta_j g_{ij} + \varepsilon_{Xi}. \tag{4.9}$$

The fitted values $\hat{x}_i = \hat{\beta}_0 + \sum_k \hat{\beta}_k g_{ik}$ are then used in the second-stage regression model:

$$y_i = \theta_0 + \theta_1 \hat{x}_i + \varepsilon_{Yi} \tag{4.10}$$

where ε_{Xi} and ε_{Yi} are independent error terms. The causal parameter of interest is θ_1. If both models are estimated by standard linear regression, both the error terms are assumed to be normally distributed.

Although estimation of the causal effect in two stages (a sequential regression method) gives the correct point estimate, the standard error from the second-stage regression (equation 4.10) is underestimated, as uncertainty from the first-stage regression is not accounted for in the second-stage regression. The use of 2SLS software is therefore recommended for estimation, as this accounts for the uncertainty [Angrist and Pischke, 2009a]. Robust standard errors are often used in practice, as estimates are sensitive to heteroscedasticity and misspecification of the equations in the model.

Although the 2SLS method above fits a linear model relating the exposure to the genetic variants (equation 4.9), this model is not required to be correctly specified for the 2SLS method to provide consistent estimates [Vansteelandt et al., 2012]. It is not necessary to make any parametric assumptions when modelling the exposure as a function of the genetic variants. A linear model is displayed above for simplicity of presentation. If the true relationship between the variants and exposure was dominant or recessive in one of the genetic variants, then greater efficiency would be obtained by correctly specifying this model. Estimates are not generally consistent under misspecification of the gene–exposure model when the model for second-stage regression (equation 4.10) is not linear in the exposure (such as is generally the case for a binary outcome).

If the genetic model for the exposure is correctly specified and all genetic variants are valid IVs, the 2SLS represents the most efficient combination of information on multiple IVs into a single causal estimate [Wooldridge, 2009a].

4.2.2   Binary outcome

The analogue of 2SLS with binary outcomes is a two-stage estimator where the second-stage $(X\text{–}Y)$ regression uses a log-linear or logistic regression model. This can be implemented using a sequential regression method by performing the two regression stages in turn (also known as two-stage predictor substitution). As in the continuous outcome case, estimates from such an approach will be overly precise, as uncertainty in the first-stage regression is not accounted for. However, this over-precision is typically slight when the standard error in the first-stage coefficients is low.

As with the ratio IV estimator, in a case-control study it is important to undertake the first-stage regression only in the controls, not the cases (Section 4.1.4). Fitted exposure values for the cases are obtained by substituting their genetic variants into the first-stage regression model.

Two-stage regression methods with non-collapsible second-stage regression models (such as logistic regression) have been criticized and called 'forbidden regressions' [Angrist and Pischke, 2009a, page 190]. This is because the non-linear model does not guarantee that the residuals from the second-stage regression are uncorrelated with the instruments [Foster, 1997]. Some researchers have recommended additionally adjusting for the first-stage residuals in the second-stage regression model, an approach known as two-stage residual inclusion. However, this is unlikely to make estimates unbiased [Cai et al., 2011], and as it is not clear what variable is represented by the first-stage residuals, it is uncertain what odds ratio is being estimated by such an approach [Burgess and Thompson, 2012]. We therefore do not recommend adjustment for the first-stage residuals in a two-stage method.

Even if the second-stage model is not collapsible, estimates from the two-stage method are unbiased under the causal null hypothesis, and so provide a valid test of the causal null hypothesis [Vansteelandt et al., 2011]. Hence Mendelian randomization investigations still provide valid causal inferences, even when there is uncertainty in the interpretation of the causal estimate.

4.3   Example: Body mass index and smoking intensity

To illustrate the ratio and two-stage least squares methods, we take data on 367 703 individuals of European ancestries from UK Biobank, a cross-sectional study of UK residents [Sudlow et al., 2015], and investigate the causal effect of body mass index (BMI) on smoking intensity, measured in pack-years, using four genetic variants that are associated with BMI at a genome-wide level of significance as IVs. A positive IV estimate would indicate that BMI is a causal risk factor for smoking behaviour, with increased BMI leading to increases in smoking intensity. We calculate the genetic associations with the exposure and outcome using linear regression assuming an additive genetic model. We then calculate the ratio estimate for each variant, and the corresponding 95% confidence intervals using the first-order and second-order formulae (equations 4.5 and 4.7), and using Fieller's theorem.

Table 4.1 shows that the ratio estimates are positive for each of the variants, although the confidence intervals all overlap the null. The 95% confidence intervals are similar when using the first-order and second-order formulae. While this is not a universal finding, this will generally be the case when the genetic associations with the exposure are precisely estimated, as is the case here. The largest discrepancy is for rs3101336, where the confidence interval is 1.5% wider when using second-order weights. The confidence intervals from Fieller's theorem are also broadly similar. This suggests that choice of method for calculating confidence intervals is not critical in this example.

The estimate from the 2SLS method is 0.127. This represents the increase in cigarettes smoked per day per 1 kg/m^2 increase in genetically-predicted BMI. The standard error calculated using the *ivpack* package in R is 0.0712. The standard error calculated from sequential regression is 0.0716. Again, ignoring the uncertainty in the genetic associations with the exposure did not lead to substantial changes in the standard error of the overall estimate (and in this case led to a slightly larger standard error – this can occur using robust regression when errors are less heteroscedastic than would be expected due to chance). More comprehensive Mendelian randomization analyses of this question using a wider range of genetic variants have suggested that there is statistical evidence to infer a positive causal effect of BMI on smoking behaviour [Taylor et al., 2018]. We return to consider this example using summarized data in Chapter 5.

SNP	Per allele change in BMI (SE)	Per allele change in smoking (SE)	Ratio estimate	95% CI (first-order)	95% CI (second-order)	95% CI (Fieller)
rs1558902	0.355 (0.011)	0.038 (0.032)	0.106	−0.073, 0.285	−0.073, 0.285	−0.073, 0.286
rs6567160	0.258 (0.013)	0.031 (0.038)	0.120	−0.166, 0.406	−0.166, 0.406	−0.167, 0.409
rs2820292	0.097 (0.011)	0.013 (0.032)	0.138	−0.514, 0.790	−0.514, 0.791	−0.525, 0.817
rs3101336	0.105 (0.011)	0.054 (0.033)	0.512	−0.093, 1.116	−0.102, 1.126	−0.093, 1.165

TABLE 4.1
Association of four SNPs with body mass index (BMI, kg/m^2 units) and smoking intensity (pack-years). Causal estimates are obtained from the ratio method, and 95% confidence intervals (CI) are calculated using three approaches: normal approximation with first-order standard errors, normal approximation with second-order standard errors, and Fieller's theorem.

4.4   Computer implementation

Several commands are available in statistical software packages for IV estimation, such as Stata [StataCorp, 2009], SAS [SAS, 2004], and R [R Development Core Team, 2011]. We assume that the reader is familiar enough with the software to perform the ratio method.

4.4.1   IV analysis of continuous outcomes in Stata

The main command in Stata to implement the 2SLS method is `ivreg2` [Baum et al., 2003]. If the exposure is x, the outcome is y and the IV is g, the syntax for a 2SLS analysis is:

```
ivreg2 y (x=g)
```

The commands `ivregress 2sls y (x=g)` and `ivreg y (x=g)` give the same estimates as `ivreg2 y (x=g)`, but a more limited output. The command `ivhettest` performs a test of heteroscedasticity of the errors in the second-stage regression. If heteroscedasticity is present, a generalized method of moments method with robust standard errors (Section 8.12) is preferred to a 2SLS analysis. The command `overid` gives more information about overidentification tests (referred to in this book as heterogeneity tests). The command `ivendog` gives more information about endogeneity tests (an endogeneity test assesses for difference between the observational and IV estimates). Each of these commands can be used with multiple instruments, for example, `ivreg2 y (x=g1 g2 g3)`.

4.4.2 IV analysis in SAS

The command `proc syslin` has been written to implement the 2SLS method in SAS:

```
proc syslin data=in 2sls;
 endogenous x;
 instruments g1 g2 g3;
 model y=x;
     run;
```

4.4.3 IV analysis in R

The `ivreg` command in the *ivpack* package has been written to implement the 2SLS method in R [Small, 2014]:

```
ivmodel.all = ivreg(y~x|g1+g2+g3, x=TRUE)
summary(ivmodel.all)
summary(ivmodel.all)$coef[2]    # 2SLS estimate
summary(ivmodel.all)$coef[2,2] # standard error of 2SLS estimate
```

In a two-stage analysis of a binary outcome in a case-control setting using logistic regression, inference on the controls only (where $Y = 0$) can be made by sequential regression using the `predict` function:

```
g0=g[y==0]
glm(y~predict(lm(x[y==0]~g0), newdata=list(g0=g)),
    family=binomial)
```

4.5 Summary

We have introduced two methods for causal estimation with individual-level data. Both the ratio and two-stage methods assume that genetic variants are all valid IVs. Each of the methods is relatively straightforward to implement, requiring nothing more complicated than regression. While there is a dazzling array of more sophisticated methods for IV analysis, the ratio and two-stage methods are foundational to the understanding of Mendelian randomization.

In the next chapter, we consider how the same estimates can be obtained using summarized data, a technique that has transformed Mendelian randomization practice by allowing a wide range of analyses to be performed quickly and easily.

5

Estimating a causal effect from summarized data

In the previous chapter, we showed that the ratio method for a single genetic variant could be performed using summarized data on genetic associations with the exposure and with the outcome. In this chapter, we introduce the inverse-variance weighted method, which combines summarized data for multiple variants into a single causal estimate. We show that estimates from the inverse-variance weighted method are the same as those obtained from the two-stage method, and hence most efficiently combine information from multiple valid instrumental variables.

5.1 Motivating example: interleukin-1 and cardiovascular diseases

In 2015, Daniel Freitag was the lead author for a Mendelian randomization paper evaluating the causal role of interleukin-1, an inflammatory marker, for various cardiovascular diseases [The Interleukin-1 Genetics Consortium, 2015]. The design of the paper was as follows. First, he demonstrated that two common variants in the *IL1RN* gene region which codes for interleukin-1 receptor antagonist (IL-1Ra) were associated with circulating levels of IL-1Ra. Secondly, he showed that the variants were inversely associated with risk of rheumatoid arthritis. This mirrors the effect of anakinra, a recombinant form of IL-1Ra that is used as a treatment for rheumatoid arthritis. The associations of the variants with downstream inflammatory markers (C-reactive protein and interleukin-6) were in the same direction as observed in patients treated with anakinra. This provides evidence that the genetic variants act in a similar way to interleukin-1 inhibition, and hence genetic associations with outcomes should reflect the predicted impact of interleukin-1 inhibition.

Figure 5.1 shows the genetic associations with risk of rheumatoid arthritis, Type 2 diabetes, coronary heart disease (CHD), ischaemic stroke, and abdominal aortic aneurysm. These associations suggest that while interleukin-1 inhibition reduces the risk of rheumatoid arthritis, it increases the risk of coronary heart disease and abdominal aortic aneurysm.

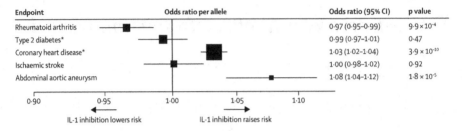

FIGURE 5.1
Mendelian randomization estimates for interleukin-1. Estimates represent odds ratios per interleukin-1 receptor antagonist increasing allele. Error bars represent 95% confidence intervals. Taken from The Interleukin-1 Genetics Consortium [2015].

Aside from this being an elegant example of Mendelian randomization in practice, we present this example to explain the value of summarized data and the need for methods that combine data on multiple genetic variants. In order to compile the Mendelian randomization estimates in Figure 5.1, Daniel Freitag had to write to around thirty different studies to request data. This process took around two years and over a thousand emails. Nowadays, meta-analysed genetic association estimates have been made publicly available for download by several large genetic consortia. Data gathering for hundreds of disease outcomes can be done at the touch of a button. Summarized data allow these analyses to be performed quickly and efficiently, enabling wide-ranging Mendelian randomization investigations to be performed for a large number of outcomes with relative ease.

As an additional point, at the time of the investigation, neither of the two genetic variants in the *IL1RN* gene region was associated with CHD risk at a genome-wide level of significance. However, when combining the evidence on the two variants together, a genome-wide level of significance was achieved for the combined analysis. This motivates the development of the inverse-variance weighted method, a method for efficiently combining summarized data on genetic associations into a single causal estimate.

5.2 Inverse-variance weighted method

We initially assume that the exposure and outcome are continuous, and return to the binary outcome case later (Section 5.2.7).

5.2.1 Summarized data on genetic associations

We assume that there are J genetic variants that are valid instrumental variables (IVs), the effect of the exposure on the outcome is linear with no effect modification, and the associations of the genetic variants with the exposure and with the outcome are linear without effect modification. The model relating the variables is:

$$\mathbb{E}(X|G_j = g, U = u) = \beta_{X0j} + \beta_{Xj}\, g + \beta_{XU}\, u \tag{5.1}$$
$$\mathbb{E}(Y|G_j = g, U = u) = \beta_{Y0j} + \beta_{Yj}\, g + \beta_{YU}\, u \quad \text{for } j = 1, \dots, J$$
$$\mathbb{E}(Y|do(X = x), U = u) = \theta_0 + \theta\, x + \beta_U\, u$$

where X is the exposure, $G_1, \dots, G_J$ are the genetic variants, Y is the outcome, U is an unmeasured confounder, $do(X = x)$ is Pearl's do-operator meaning that the value of the exposure is set to x by intervention [Pearl, 2000a], and the causal effect parameter $\theta = \frac{\beta_{Yj}}{\beta_{Xj}}$ for all $j = 1, \dots, J$. This means that the ratio estimates for each genetic variant are consistent estimates of the same causal parameter. We return to the case where this is not true later (Section 5.3).

In this notation, the ratio estimate based on the jth genetic variant is:

$$\hat{\theta}_j = \frac{\hat{\beta}_{Yj}}{\hat{\beta}_{Xj}} \tag{5.2}$$

and its approximate standard error is:

$$\text{se}(\hat{\theta}_j) = |\frac{\text{se}(\hat{\beta}_{Yj})}{\hat{\beta}_{Xj}}|, \tag{5.3}$$

where hats indicate that the quantities are estimated and the vertical lines indicate taking the positive value of the expression. This is the first-order standard error estimate, which we assume is a reasonable representation of the uncertainty in the ratio estimate. It only takes into account the uncertainty in the genetic association with the outcome, but this is typically much greater than the uncertainty in the genetic association with the exposure (particularly if the variant is associated with the exposure at a genome-wide level of significance).

The $\hat{\beta}_{Xj}$ and $\hat{\beta}_{Yj}$ association estimates and their respective standard errors $\text{se}(\hat{\beta}_{Xj})$ and $\text{se}(\hat{\beta}_{Yj})$ are referred to as summarized data. They are obtained from regression of the exposure or outcome on each genetic variant in turn. Although the models in equation (5.1) are conditional on the confounder U, G_j is independent of U since it is a valid IV, and hence the same quantity is estimated even when we do not adjust for U. In practice, genetic associations are often adjusted for principal components of ancestry to avoid bias due to population stratification (see Section 8.6 for a fuller discussion on covariate adjustment).

We refer to the ratio estimate $\hat{\theta}_j$ as a variant-specific causal estimate, as it is only calculated using information on variant j. Generally it is not important which allele the genetic associations are reported with respect to (that is, the minor allele or the major allele), provided the associations with the exposure and outcome are both reported with respect to the same allele. We refer to this as the 'effect allele' and the other allele as the 'reference allele'. Switching the effect allele would change the signs of the associations from positive to negative (or vice versa); this would not change the ratio estimate for that variant (as the numerator and denominator would both switch signs).

5.2.2   Inverse-variance weighted meta-analysis

When there are multiple IVs, then a more precise estimate of the causal effect can be obtained by combining information on all the IVs into a single estimate. If individual-level data are available, the two-stage least squares (2SLS) method is performed by regressing the exposure on the instrumental variables, and then regressing the outcome on fitted values of the exposure from the first stage regression (Section 4.2.1). It is the most efficient (that is, lowest variance) unbiased combination of the variant-specific estimates [Wooldridge, 2009a].

The inverse-variance weighted (IVW) method is motivated as a meta-analysis of the variant-specific causal estimates. If we have several independent estimates of the same quantity, the most efficient way of combining them into a single estimate is an inverse-variance weighted meta-analysis [Borenstein et al., 2009]. If the genetic variants are uncorrelated, then their genetic associations will be uncorrelated in large samples. The IVW estimate can be expressed as:

$$\hat{\theta}_{IVW} = \frac{\sum_j \hat{\theta}_j \, \mathrm{se}(\hat{\theta}_j)^{-2}}{\sum_j \mathrm{se}(\hat{\theta}_j)^{-2}} \tag{5.4}$$

$$= \frac{\sum_j \hat{\beta}_{Yj} \hat{\beta}_{Xj} \, \mathrm{se}(\hat{\beta}_{Yj})^{-2}}{\sum_j \hat{\beta}_{Xj}{}^2 \, \mathrm{se}(\hat{\beta}_{Yj})^{-2}}.$$

This is a weighted average (or, more formally, a weighted mean) of the variant-specific causal estimates. The (fixed-effect) standard error of the IVW estimate is:

$$\mathrm{se}(\hat{\theta}_{IVW}) = \sqrt{\frac{1}{\sum_j \hat{\beta}_{Xj}{}^2 \, \mathrm{se}(\hat{\beta}_{Yj})^{-2}}}. \tag{5.5}$$

This is the form of the inverse-variance weighted estimate as it was initially proposed [The International Consortium for Blood Pressure Genome-Wide Association Studies, 2011; Dastani et al., 2012; Johnson, 2013]. While these formulae may look complicated, they only require the multiplication and addition of numbers (and one square root), and could in principle be calculated using a pocket calculator.

5.2.3 Weighted linear regression

The IVW estimate can also be obtained by weighted regression using the following model:

$$\hat{\beta}_{Yj} = \theta\,\hat{\beta}_{Xj} + \varepsilon_j, \quad \varepsilon_j \sim \mathcal{N}(0, \mathrm{se}(\hat{\beta}_{Yj})^2). \tag{5.6}$$

This is a weighted linear regression with no intercept term, in which the slope parameter is the causal estimate, and the weights are the reciprocals of the variances of the genetic associations with the outcome $\mathrm{se}(\hat{\beta}_{Yj})^{-2}$. The estimated slope parameter is equal to the IVW estimate [Burgess et al., 2016c].

5.2.4 Equivalence to two-stage least squares estimate

The IVW estimate using first-order weights is also equal to the estimate obtained from the 2SLS method that is commonly used with individual-level data (sample size N). If we write the exposure as X ($N \times 1$ matrix), the outcome as Y ($N \times 1$ matrix), and the instrumental variables as G ($N \times J$ matrix), then the 2SLS estimate is:

$$\hat{\theta}_{2SLS} = [X^T G (G^T G)^{-1} G^T X]^{-1} X^T G (G^T G)^{-1} G^T Y.$$

Regression of Y on G gives beta-coefficients $\hat{\beta}_Y = (G^T G)^{-1} G^T Y$ with standard errors the square roots of the diagonal elements of the matrix $(G^T G)^{-1} \sigma^2$ where σ is the residual standard error. If the instrumental variables are perfectly uncorrelated, then the off-diagonal elements of $(G^T G)^{-1} \sigma^2$ are all equal to zero. Regression of X on G gives beta-coefficients $\hat{\beta}_X = (G^T G)^{-1} G^T X$. Weighted linear regression of the beta-coefficients $\hat{\beta}_Y$ on the beta-coefficients $\hat{\beta}_X$ using the inverse-variance weights $(G^T G)\sigma^{-2}$ gives an estimate:

$$[\hat{\beta}_X^T (G^T G)\hat{\beta}_X]^{-1} \sigma^{-2} \hat{\beta}_X^T (G^T G)\sigma^2 \hat{\beta}_Y$$

$$= [X^T G (G^T G)^{-1}(G^T G)(G^T G)^{-1} G^T X]^{-1} X^T G (G^T G)^{-1}(G^T G)(G^T G)^{-1} G^T Y$$

$$= [X^T G (G^T G)^{-1} G^T X]^{-1} X^T G (G^T G)^{-1} G^T Y$$

$$= \hat{\theta}_{2SLS}$$

The assumption of uncorrelated IVs ensures that the summarized data from univariate regressions on each variant in turn equal those from multivariable regression on all the variants in a single model (as in the two-stage least squares method). In practice, the two-stage least squares and weighted regression-based estimates will differ slightly as there will be non-zero correlations between the genetic variants in finite samples, even if the variants are truly uncorrelated in the population. However, these differences are likely to be slight.

5.2.5   Choice of weights

Assuming that the genetic associations with the exposure and with the outcome are independently distributed (which is the case if they are estimated in separate datasets, a two-sample analysis), the second-order standard error of the jth ratio estimate (equation 4.7) can be written using the notation of this chapter as:

$$\mathrm{se}(\hat{\theta}_j) = \sqrt{\frac{\mathrm{se}(\hat{\beta}_{Yj})^2}{\hat{\beta}_{Xj}{}^2} + \frac{\hat{\beta}_{Yj}{}^2\,\mathrm{se}(\hat{\beta}_{Xj})^2}{\hat{\beta}_{Xj}{}^4}}. \tag{5.7}$$

While the use of second-order standard errors to form the weights in calculating the IVW estimate is possible, and seems appealing, the second-order weights depend on the genetic associations with the outcome $\hat{\beta}_{Yj}$, leading to a correlation between the jth ratio estimate and its standard error. This can lead to the IVW method based on second-order weights having worse properties in practice [Thompson et al., 2016; Bowden et al., 2019]. A solution for using modified weights that allows for the uncertainty in the genetic associations with the exposure has been proposed [Bowden et al., 2019]. However, the use of first-order standard errors is often reasonable in practice.

5.2.6   Correlated variants

If the genetic variants are correlated, then performing a meta-analysis of the variant-specific estimates ignoring this correlation is inappropriate. Meta-analyses of estimates from two perfectly correlated variants is equivalent to double-counting the data. The correlations between variant-specific estimates will be approximately equal to the correlations between the variants themselves [Verzilli et al., 2008]. This means that correlations can be estimated from reference data on individuals from the same population group as the sample under investigation.

We can perform the IVW method with correlated genetic variants by weighted generalized linear regression of the $\hat{\beta}_{Yj}$ estimates on the $\hat{\beta}_{Xj}$ estimates. We note that these are still the coefficients from regression on each variant in turn. With correlated variants, these marginal associations would differ from the conditional associations obtained from regression on all variants in a single model; it is the marginal associations that are required for the IVW method.

If $\rho_{j_1 j_2}$ is the correlation between variants j_1 and j_2, and Ω is a matrix with elements $\Omega_{j_1 j_2} = \text{se}(\hat{\beta}_{Y j_1}) \, \text{se}(\hat{\beta}_{Y j_2}) \rho_{j_1 j_2}$, then our regression model is:

$$\hat{\boldsymbol{\beta}}_Y = \theta \, \hat{\boldsymbol{\beta}}_X + \boldsymbol{\varepsilon}, \quad \boldsymbol{\varepsilon} \sim \mathcal{N}(\mathbf{0}, \Omega). \tag{5.8}$$

where bold face represents vectors and the error distribution is multivariable normal. The estimate from a weighted generalized linear regression is:

$$\hat{\theta}_{IVW,c} = (\hat{\boldsymbol{\beta}}_X^T \Omega^{-1} \hat{\boldsymbol{\beta}}_X)^{-1} \hat{\boldsymbol{\beta}}_X^T \Omega^{-1} \hat{\boldsymbol{\beta}}_Y. \tag{5.9}$$

The (fixed-effect) standard error of the estimate is:

$$\text{se}(\hat{\theta}_{IVW,c}) = \sqrt{(\hat{\boldsymbol{\beta}}_X^T \Omega^{-1} \hat{\boldsymbol{\beta}}_X)^{-1}}. \tag{5.10}$$

This estimate is also equivalent to the 2SLS estimate with correlated variants.

Inclusion of genetic variants that are perfectly correlated will not result in gains in efficiency for the IVW estimate. Inclusion of partially correlated variants will improve efficiency if the extra variants explain additional variation in the exposure. This is equivalent to saying that they are conditionally associated with the exposure in a multivariable regression model. Some caution is required though: if large numbers of correlated variants are included in an analysis, then small discrepancies in correlation estimates can lead to overly precise estimates [Burgess et al., 2017c].

5.2.7 Binary outcomes

As with the ratio and two-stage methods for individual-level data, the IVW method can be performed with a binary outcome. We replace the linearity assumptions for the genetic associations with the outcome and the structural model for the relationship between the exposure and outcome with log-linear or logistic models. If the genetic association estimates for the outcome are estimated using a log-linear or logistic regression model, then the resulting IVW estimate is equivalent to the relevant log-linear or logistic two-stage estimate. For a log-linear model, the IVW estimate represents a causal log risk ratio. For a logistic regression model, the IVW estimate represents a causal log odds ratio, but there are issues of interpretation due to the non-collapsibility of the odds ratio (Section 8.7). As for the two-stage method (Section 4.2.2), even for a non-collapsible measure, the IVW estimate is a valid estimate under the causal null hypothesis, and so represents a valid test statistic for the causal null hypothesis.

5.3   Heterogeneity and pleiotropy

Even if the IV assumptions are satisfied for each genetic variant, it is plausible that the variant-specific ratio estimates $\hat{\theta}_j$ differ by more than expected due to chance alone. This could occur for a number of reasons: both statistical and biological. Statistical reasons include non-linearity, departure from the homogeneity assumption, and different complier populations under the monotonicity assumption. Also, different genetic variants may be associated with different trajectories of change in the exposure over time even if the instantaneous associations at the time of measurement are equal. Biological reasons include that the exposure is not a single entity, but in fact contains multiple components with distinct causal effects, and that the exposure can be intervened on in different ways, with each intervention leading to a different size of change in the outcome. For example, interventions to lower BMI via decreasing an individual's caloric intake may lead to less cardiovascular benefit compared with interventions to increase metabolic rate.

However, differences between the variant-specific ratio estimates that are greater than expected by chance alone may also occur because one or more variants are not valid IVs. For example, in a Mendelian randomization analysis of low-density lipoprotein (LDL) cholesterol on risk of Alzheimer's disease, genetic associations are close to zero for the majority of variants, and only differ from zero for two variants (Figure 5.2). The likely explanation is that LDL-cholesterol is not a causal risk factor for Alzheimer's disease, and these two variants (which are both in the *APOE* gene region) are pleiotropic.

Heterogeneity between the variant-specific causal estimates can be assessed using techniques from meta-analysis. Visual plotting of the summarized association estimates can be helpful to identify outliers. In fact, even when the analyst has access to individual-level data, we would recommend calculating summarized associations so that variant-specific estimates can be compared visually. In addition to the scatter plot illustrated in Figure 5.2, funnel plots [Burgess et al., 2017a], and radial plots [Bowden et al., 2018b] are useful tools for exploring heterogeneity and identifying outliers, which may represent invalid IVs.

There are also statistical approaches for measuring heterogeneity. For example, Cochran's Q statistic can be calculated. This is a weighted sum of the squared distances of the variant-specific estimates from the overall IVW estimate:

$$Q = \sum_j \text{se}(\hat{\theta}_j)^{-2}(\hat{\theta}_{IVW} - \hat{\theta}_j)^2$$

Under the null hypothesis that each variant identifies the same causal parameter, this approximately has a chi-squared distribution on $J-1$ degrees of freedom, where J is the number of genetic variants [Greco et al., 2015]. A large value of the Q statistic means that the variant-specific ratio estimates

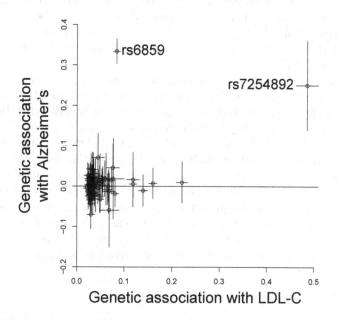

FIGURE 5.2

Genetic associations with LDL-cholesterol (horizontal axis, standard deviation units) and with Alzheimer's disease (vertical axis, log odds ratios) for 75 genetic variants associated with LDL-cholesterol at a genome-wide level of significance. Lines represent 95% confidence intervals for the genetic associations. Most points suggest a null causal effect. The two marked outlying variants suggest a positive causal effect, but these are likely to be pleiotropic and hence unreliable. Taken from Rees et al. [2019b].

differ by more than expected due to chance alone. In econometrics, an equivalent test is known as an overidentification test. With individual-level data, this can be undertaken by testing for association between the IVs and the residual term in the second-stage of the 2SLS method. Under the null hypothesis of homogeneity, the residual term should not be associated with the IVs. Higgins I^2 statistic can also be used to quantify the degree of heterogeneity [Higgins et al., 2003]. This is important when large numbers of variants are included in an analysis, as the Q statistic may reject the null hypothesis of homogeneity even though the amount of heterogeneity is small. Individual outliers and influential points can also be identified when implementing the IVW method by weighted regression using standard regression diagnostics such as Studentized residuals and Cook's distances [Corbin et al., 2016].

If there is evidence of heterogeneity, we would urge caution in the interpretation of both the heterogeneity result and the Mendelian randomization investigation. If heterogeneity is due to distinct outliers that contribute the vast majority of the heterogeneity, then these may be isolated invalid IVs. Of course, the opposite could be true, and the majority of variants may be invalid and the outliers valid. But it is implausible that a large number of genetic variants are invalid in the same way leading to similar variant-specific estimates. Alternatively, if estimates are more dispersed than would be expected by chance, but the burden of overdispersion is shared across several of the variants, then it may simply be that different variants affect the exposure in different ways, but there are no invalid IVs. Hence while heterogeneity is a cause for concern, in isolation it should not invalidate findings.

5.3.1   Fixed- and random-effects models

The use of random-effects models is a practical step to address heterogeneity by decreasing the precision of estimates when heterogeneity is detected. A fixed-effect model assumes that the variant-specific estimates all target the same causal parameter. A random-effects model allows for variation in the causal parameters targeted by the variants. Although random-effects models in the meta-analysis literature are typically performed using an additive model, we advocate multiplicative random-effects models for Mendelian randomization.

In an additive random-effects model, the variant-specific estimands are assumed to be normally distributed with variance ϕ_A^2. An estimand is the quantity targeted by an estimate. This means that there are two sources of variability in the variant-specific estimates: the variance $\text{se}(\hat{\theta}_j)^2$ owing to imprecision in the estimate, and the heterogeneity ϕ_A^2 owing to differences in the quantities targeted. In an additive model, the overall variance used in the weighting of the IVW estimate is a sum of these two terms. In a multiplicative random-effects model, the variant-specific estimates are assumed to be normally distributed with variance $\phi_M^2 \, \text{se}(\hat{\theta}_j)^2$, where ϕ_M^2 is an overdispersion parameter:

$$\hat{\beta}_{Yj} = \theta\,\hat{\beta}_{Xj} + \varepsilon_j, \quad \varepsilon_j \sim \mathcal{N}(0, \phi_M^2\,\mathrm{se}(\hat{\beta}_{Yj})^2). \tag{5.11}$$

A multiplicative random-effects model can be implemented by allowing the residual standard error in the regression model to be estimated. In a fixed-effect analysis, this parameter is fixed to be one [Thompson and Sharp, 1999], but in a multiplicative random-effects analysis, we allow this term (which represents overdispersion of the variance-specific causal estimates) to be estimated. We do not allow it to take values less than one, as underdispersion is statistically and biologically implausible, so we take its value as the maximum of the estimated value and 1. In a multiplicative random-effects model, the standard error of the IVW estimate is:

$$\mathrm{se}(\hat{\theta}_{IVW}) = \frac{\hat{\phi}_M^*}{\sqrt{\sum_j \hat{\beta}_{Xj}^2\,\mathrm{se}(\hat{\beta}_{Yj})^{-2}}}. \tag{5.12}$$

where $\hat{\phi}_M^* = \max(1, \hat{\phi}_M)$ and $\hat{\phi}_M$ is the estimate of the residual standard error.

There are two main reasons why we prefer a multiplicative to an additive random-effects model. First, the point estimates from the fixed-effect and multiplicative random-effects are identical. Using a random-effects model widens confidence intervals in the case of heterogeneity, but otherwise results remain the same. Secondly, a multiplicative random-effects model does not change the relative weights of the estimates in the meta-analysis. If there is heterogeneity, an additive random-effects model reduces the weight assigned to the most precise estimates and shares the weight more evenly amongst all estimates. This has been criticized in the field of meta-analysis, as more precise estimates are generally more reliable. A further reason is that the IVW estimate (fixed-effect and multiplicative random-effects) is a consistent estimate under the assumption of balanced pleiotropy, defined in Section 7.4.1.

Unless there is good reason for believing that all variants target the same parameter (for example, because all variants are from a single gene region, or there are very few variants in the analysis so heterogeneity cannot be estimated reliably), we would generally advocate random-effects models for Mendelian randomization. If there is no excess heterogeneity in the variant-specific causal estimates, then the random-effects and fixed-effect results will be identical, so there is no loss of precision. If there is excess heterogeneity in the variant-specific causal estimates, then the fixed-effect estimate is overly precise, and this heterogeneity should be accounted for. If there is statistical evidence for a causal effect in a random-effects analysis, this means that there is consistent evidence that the genetic variants support a causal effect of the exposure on the outcome even accounting for heterogeneity in the variant-specific causal estimates.

5.4   Computer implementation

The inverse-variance weighted method is implemented for R in the `mr_ivw`
command in the *MendelianRandomization* package available from the
Comprehensive R Archive Network (CRAN) [Yavorska and Burgess, 2017].
The syntax is:

```
mr_ivw(mr_input(bx, bxse, by, byse))
```

where `bx` and `by` are the genetic associations with the exposure and outcome,
and `bxse` and `byse` are their standard errors. A multiplicative random-effects
model is chosen by default when the number of variants is four or more. The
function automatically reports a heterogeneity test based on Cochran's Q
statistic. The IVW estimate can also be obtained by direct calculation:

```
sum(by*bx*byse^-2)/sum(bx^2*byse^-2)
```

or by meta-analysis:

```
library(meta)
metagen(by/bx, abs(byse/bx))$TE.fixed
```

or by weighted regression:

```
lm(by~bx-1, weights=byse^-2)$coef[1]
```

However, standard errors from these commands are not guaranteed to be
correct. The `metagen` command allows the user to obtain a standard error
corresponding to either a fixed-effect or an additive random-effects model.
Standard errors from the `lm` command correspond to a multiplicative random-
effects model, except that there is no prohibition on underdispersion, meaning
that the reported standard error may be lower than that from a fixed-effect
analysis. A corrected standard error from a multiplicative random-effects
model can be obtained by dividing by the minimum of the estimated residual
standard error and 1:

```
summary(lm(by~bx-1, weights=byse^-2))$coef[1,2]/
  min(summary(lm(by~bx-1, weights=byse^-2))$sigma, 1)
```

We therefore recommend the `mr_ivw` command for use in practice.
  The `mr_ivw` command can incorporate correlated variants:

```
mr_ivw(mr_input(bx, bxse, by, byse, correlation=rho))
```

where `rho` is the correlation matrix. The *MendelianRandomization* package
contains many other useful commands, such as the `mr_plot` command for
drawing an interactive scatter plot of the summarized data.

A similar function, also called mr_ivw, is available in the *TwoSampleMR* package, available from https://mrcieu.github.io/TwoSampleMR/ [Hemani et al., 2018b]. This package also has a function ld_matrix, which calculates a correlation matrix between variants from reference data.

The inverse-variance weighted method is implemented for Stata in the *mrrobust* package [Spiller et al., 2019].

5.4.1 Finding summarized genetic association data

Several sources of summarized genetic association data are available from various consortia via supplementary tables and material of published papers, and via dedicated download sites. Two particular resources that have aggregated summarized data are PhenoScanner (http://www.phenoscanner. medschl.cam.ac.uk/) [Staley et al., 2016; Kamat et al., 2019], and MR-Base (http://www.mrbase.org/) [Hemani et al., 2018b]. Data from PhenoScanner can be obtained through seamless integration with the *MendelianRandomization* package in R. For example:

```
mr_obj = pheno_input(snps=c("rs12916", "rs2479409", "rs217434", "rs1367117"),
  exposure = "Low density lipoprotein", pmidE = "24097068", ancestryE = "European",
  outcome = "Coronary artery disease", pmidO = "26343387", ancestryO = "Mixed")
mr_ivw(mr_obj)
```

In this example, genetic associations with the exposure 'Low density lipoprotein' are obtained from a published study with PubMed ID 24097068 and estimated in a European-ancestry population, and genetic associations with the outcome 'Coronary artery disease' are obtained from a published study with PubMed ID 26343387 and estimated in a mixed-ancestry population. Specifying the name of the exposure/outcome, the PubMed ID of the reference in which the associations were published, and the ancestry group provides a unique specification in the PhenoScanner database of genetic associations. The code finds the relevant associations for the four genetic variants specified (rs12916, rs2479409, rs217434, and rs1367117) and returns an object that can be analysed by the mr_ivw command.

Mendelian randomization analyses using summarized data can therefore be performed with just a few lines of code. While this is undoubtably improves accessibility and reproducibility of investigations, it is important to remember that the difficult part of a Mendelian randomization analysis is not the computational method, but deciding what should go into the analysis. The availability of these tools should enable less attention to be paid to the mechanics of the analysis, and more attention to these choices. However, they also run the risk of encouraging large numbers of speculative analyses to be performed in an unprincipled way.

5.5   Example: Body mass index and smoking intensity reprised

Returning to the example of the effect of body mass index (BMI) on smoking intensity from Section 4.3, we show how to address this question using publicly-available summarized data. We do not make any attempt to validate the genetic variants as IVs here for brevity and to illustrate the method; any causal claim based on this analysis would be premature before the validity of the genetic variants as IVs was interrogated.

We consider 31 genetic variants previously shown to be associated with BMI at a genome-wide level of significance [Speliotes et al., 2010]. We take genetic associations with BMI (measured in standard deviation units) from the GIANT consortium [Locke et al., 2015] (the PubMed ID of the reference paper is 25673413), and genetic associations with smoking intensity (measured in cigarettes per day) from the Tobacco and Alcohol Consortium [Tobacco and Genetics Consortium, 2010] (the PubMed ID of the reference paper is 20418890). The code is as follows:

```
library(MendelianRandomization)
bmi_snps <- c("rs1558902", "rs2867125", "rs571312", "rs10938397",
 "rs10767664", "rs2815752", "rs7359397", "rs9816226", "rs3817334",
 "rs29941", "rs543874", "rs987237", "rs7138803", "rs10150332",
 "rs713586", "rs12444979", "rs2241423", "rs2287019", "rs1514175",
 "rs13107325", "rs2112347", "rs10968576", "rs3810291", "rs887912",
 "rs13078807", "rs11847697", "rs2890652", "rs1555543", "rs4771122",
 "rs4836133", "rs4929949", "rs206936")
mr_obj = pheno_input(bmi_snps,
 exposure="Body mass index", pmidE="25673413", ancestryE="European",
 outcome="Cigarettes per day", pmidO="20418890", ancestryO="European")
mr_ivw(mr_obj)
mr_plot(mr_obj, interactive=FALSE, orientate=TRUE)
```

Genetic associations are displayed in Figure 5.3. The IVW estimate is 1.465 with standard error 0.490 (p-value 0.003). This represents the increase in cigarettes smoked per day per 1 standard deviation increase in genetically-predicted BMI. While there is no single variant that is strongly associated with the outcome, it is clear that the overall trend is towards a positive association with the outcome. The IVW estimate indicates that there is statistical evidence that this trend is stronger than would be expected purely by chance. There are no clear outliers on the scatter plot, and the Q statistic for heterogeneity is 27.3 (p-value 0.61 compared to a χ^2_{30} distribution), so there is no more heterogeneity between the variant-specific estimates than expected due to chance alone.

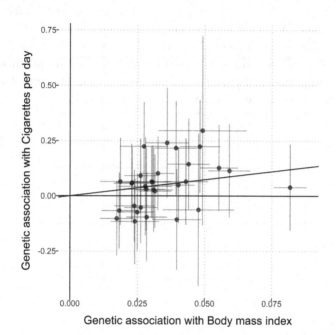

FIGURE 5.3
Genetic associations with body mass index (horizontal axis, standard deviation units) and with smoking intensity (vertical axis, cigarettes per day) for 31 genetic variants associated with body mass index at a genome-wide level of significance. Horizontal and vertical lines represent 95% confidence intervals for the genetic associations, and the line through the origin represents the IVW estimate. This graph was produced using the `mr_plot` command from the *MendelianRandomization* software package for R.

5.6   Summary

In summary, the inverse-variance weighted method combines summarized
data on multiple genetic variants to provide an estimate equal to that
which would have been obtained from a two-stage method if individual-
level data were available. This has allowed the widespread proliferation of
Mendelian randomization analyses using publicly-available data. However, the
inverse-variance weighted method assumes that all genetic variants are valid
instrumental variables, an assumption that may not hold in practice. Before
considering approaches that challenge this assumption, we next discuss the
interpretation of estimates from Mendelian randomization.

6

Interpretation of estimates from Mendelian randomization

In the previous chapters, we have introduced definitions of causal concepts and presented methods and examples of causal effects estimated using genetic variants as instrumental variables. In this chapter, we consider the interpretation of causal effects assessed and estimated in Mendelian randomization, and address the question of under what circumstances a Mendelian randomization estimate may be a reliable guide to the effect of an intervention on the exposure of interest in practice.

6.1 Internal and external validity

From the first discussions of Mendelian randomization, researchers have emphasized that the assumptions leading to the assertion of a causal relationship may be invalid for many genetic variants. Violations in the assumptions of no direct effect of the genetic variant on the outcome or of no association with a confounding risk factor may occur for several reasons, as discussed in Chapter 3. Such violations of internal validity can potentially lead to misleading conclusions. An aspect of Mendelian randomization which is less well appreciated is the issue of external validity. If the instrumental variable (IV) assumptions about the genetic variant are true and a valid estimate is made which corresponds to a causal effect, what questions are raised in interpreting this estimate in a practical context? For example, is the estimate of lowered risk derived from considering genetically lower levels of blood pressure the same as the risk reduction conferred by a clinical intervention that reduces blood pressure?

Mendelian randomization differs from a randomized trial in a fundamental way which impacts on questions of external validity [Rothwell, 2010]. In a randomized trial, the intervention applied to the treatment group is usually identical or similar to the intervention which is proposed to be applied in clinical practice. In Mendelian randomization, the 'intervention' leading to differences between genetically-defined subgroups within the study is the presence of a genetic variant. The question of external validity is whether the causal effect due to the change in the exposure as a result of the presence of the genetic variant is similar to the causal effect due to the proposed intervention on the exposure. There are several reasons why these effects may be unequal, as we now discuss.

6.1.1   Time-scale and developmental compensation

First, the presence or absence of the genetic variant in an individual is determined at conception. This means that the Mendelian randomization estimate represents the result of a life-long difference in the exposure between the genetic subgroups [Davey Smith, 2006]. In many cases, the benefit of a clinical intervention depends on the cumulative exposure to a particular risk factor over time. For example, trials have shown that the benefit of taking statins for one year is around a 10% relative reduction in coronary heart disease risk, increasing in a dose-dependent way to around 25% for five years on statins [Ference et al., 2012]. A Mendelian randomization estimate represents the impact of an even longer change in the exposure – typically, a life-long change.

Further, most clinical interventions are performed on mature individuals. It may be that a stage of disease progression is irreversible. Alternatively, an individual may develop compensatory mechanisms in response to long-term elevated (or lowered) levels of the exposure, known as canalization (Section 3.2.3). There may be no intervention on the exposure in a mature cohort which can imitate the genetic effect. This may be especially relevant if the genetic change in the exposure affects intra-uterine or early-stage development. A plausible example here is vitamin D as a risk factor for multiple sclerosis. Studies of migrants have suggested that exposure to vitamin D in early childhood is critical to reduce disease risk [Gale and Martyn, 1995]. Hence, even though Mendelian randomization studies provide evidence that vitamin D is a causal risk factor for multiple sclerosis [Mokry et al., 2015], vitamin D supplementation in adults may not reduce disease risk.

6.1.2   Usual versus pathological levels

Secondly, the genetic variant would be expected to affect average or 'usual' levels of the exposure. This is often the target of interest for epidemiologists interested in disease prevention. Mendelian randomization has a particular role to play here, as life-long randomized trials affecting usual levels of exposures cannot easily be undertaken. However, Mendelian randomization studies are unlikely to be informative about the acute response behaviour of an individual to a stimulus, such as a sudden large increase in an inflammation biomarker. It is plausible that long-term elevated average levels of an exposure for an individual do not affect the outcome, but acute response of the exposure does. The efficacy of short-term targeted interventions on pathological levels of an exposure cannot be assessed by a Mendelian randomization approach.

An example is that of C-reactive protein (CRP). Genetic variants which are associated with usual levels of CRP have been used to assess the causal effect of long-term elevated average levels of CRP on cardiovascular risk [Elliott et al., 2009; CCGC, 2011]. Although the causal effect of CRP on cardiovascular risk appears to be null, this does not preclude the efficacy of a therapeutic intervention on acute levels of CRP.

6.1.3 Extrapolation of small differences

Thirdly, changes in an exposure due to genetic variants are generally small. For evolutionary reasons, genetic variants associated with substantial changes in clinically relevant exposures are uncommon. Several sets of genetic variants which have been used in Mendelian randomization studies have explained in the region of 1 to 4% of the variation in the exposure [Schatzkin et al., 2009; Davey Smith, 2011]. If the target of interest for the epidemiologist is an intervention lowering (or raising) the exposure uniformly by a small amount for everyone in the population, then a Mendelian randomization study may provide a relevant estimate of the effect of the intervention. However, if the proposed intervention effect is more substantial, then the Mendelian randomization estimate relies on extrapolation beyond the genetic change in the exposure observed. Estimates relying on a linear assumption for the effect of the exposure on the outcome may not be valid; moreover this assumption may not be testable from empirical data.

6.1.4 Different pathways of genetic and intervention effects

Fourthly, the genetic variant and the proposed intervention will not always have the same specific mechanism of effect on the exposure. The genetic change in the exposure may operate by a causal pathway via another variable. For example, variants in the *FTO* gene influence body mass index (BMI) by affecting satiety, which in turn affects BMI [Wardle et al., 2008]. An intervention on BMI which is not based on reducing food intake may have a different effect on the outcome to the estimate from a Mendelian randomization study using a variant in the *FTO* gene as an IV.

Equivalently, the effect of the intervention may not be limited to the exposure of interest. For example, bariatric surgery aimed at reducing BMI may also result in dietary and lifestyle changes. It is difficult to assess which changes in covariates are a direct result of a decrease in BMI and so are on the causal pathway from BMI to disease, and which are separate consequences of the intervention.

6.1.5   Differences in populations

Fifthly, genetic variants typically affect all individuals in a population. If the proposed intervention is to be made across the whole population, then Mendelian randomization using a population-based cohort may give a valid estimate of its potential effect. However, if the intervention is intended to be made in a particular subpopulation, it may not be possible to choose a cohort for a Mendelian randomization study which would give a relevant estimate. For example, an intervention on blood pressure may only be applied to those with clinically-determined hypertension, whereas a genetic variant associated with blood pressure would potentially affect the whole population.

6.2   Comparison of estimates

We here give some examples to illustrate the differences between Mendelian randomization estimates and those from other epidemiological approaches, such as effect estimates from randomized controlled trials (RCTs) and observational associations from multivariable adjusted regression models.

6.2.1   LDL-cholesterol and coronary heart disease

Coronary heart disease (CHD) is the result of a build-up of atheromatous plaques in the coronary arteries. A major component of such plaques is cholesterol, and low-density lipoprotein (LDL) cholesterol is an established causal risk factor for CHD. We here use published literature to assess the magnitude of the effect of LDL-cholesterol on CHD risk as estimated from Mendelian randomization, and from RCTs where statin drugs have been used as a clinical intervention to lower LDL-cholesterol.

A meta-analysis of genome-wide association studies reported five SNPs associated with LDL-cholesterol, but not with high-density lipoprotein (HDL) cholesterol, nor with triglycerides [Waterworth et al., 2010]. Table 6.1 gives the

SNPs and relevant genes, the estimates of association of each SNP with log-transformed LDL-cholesterol and risk of CHD, and estimates using each SNP of the causal odds ratio of CHD per 30% decrease in LDL-cholesterol using the ratio method (Section 4.1). We note that this relies on a log-linear assumption of the effect of log(LDL-cholesterol) on the odds of CHD, and between eight- and 20-fold extrapolation of the genetic effects on log(LDL-cholesterol). Although further SNPs associated with LDL-cholesterol are known, these five were chosen as they represent variants with known strong associations with LDL-cholesterol, where there is some biological knowledge to justify the assumption of the specific effect of the SNP on LDL-cholesterol. There is a dose–response relationship in the genetic associations with LDL-cholesterol and with CHD risk; this gives plausibility that LDL-cholesterol is a causal risk factor for CHD risk (Figure 6.1).

SNP (relevant gene)	Per allele change in log(LDL-C) (SE)	Per allele odds ratio of CHD (95% CI)	Odds ratio of CHD per 30% decrease in LDL-C (95% CI) [1]
rs11206510 (*PCSK9*)	0.026 (0.004)	1.07 (1.01–1.13)	0.40 (0.15–0.85)
rs660240 (*SORT1*)	−0.044 (0.004)	0.85 (0.80–0.90)	0.27 (0.15–0.44)
rs515135 (*APOB*)	−0.038 (0.004)	0.90 (0.85–0.96)	0.37 (0.19–0.66)
rs12916 (*HMGCR*)	−0.023 (0.003)	0.94 (0.90–0.99)	0.38 (0.16–0.80)
rs2738459 (*LDLR*)	−0.018 (0.004)	0.96 (0.89–1.03)	0.45 (0.07–1.95)

TABLE 6.1
Association of five SNPs with log-transformed low-density lipoprotein cholesterol (LDL-C) and coronary heart disease (CHD) risk. Causal estimates of odds ratio for 30% reduction in LDL-C on coronary heart disease from Mendelian randomization using each SNP in turn.

---

[1] A 30% decrease in LDL-C is equivalent to a change in log(LDL-C) of −0.357.

Odds ratio estimates for each SNP individually range from 0.27 to 0.45. If we assume that the five estimates of causal effect in Table 6.1 are independent, then the inverse-variance weighted method gives a combined odds ratio of 0.33 (95% CI 0.24 to 0.46) [Thompson et al., 2005].

In comparison, RCTs of statins have given lesser estimates of the benefits of reducing LDL-cholesterol levels. A meta-analysis of 9 trials of the effect of statin use on CHD comprising 69 139 participants with 6406 CHD events gave a relative risk of 0.73 (95% CI 0.70 to 0.77) based on a reduction of around 30% in LDL-cholesterol over an average follow-up time of at least three years [Cheung et al., 2004]. A more focused meta-analysis examining the effect of statin use for primary disease prevention, comprising around 27 969 individuals without a history of coronary heart disease with 1677 events, gave a similar relative risk of 0.72 (95% CI 0.65 to 0.79) over 1.5 to three years' follow-up [Taylor et al., 2013]. The data on the genetic variants, together with the combined Mendelian randomization estimate and the proportional estimate of the effect of statins (assuming the relative risk of 0.73 approximates an odds ratio of the same magnitude) are displayed in Figure 6.1.

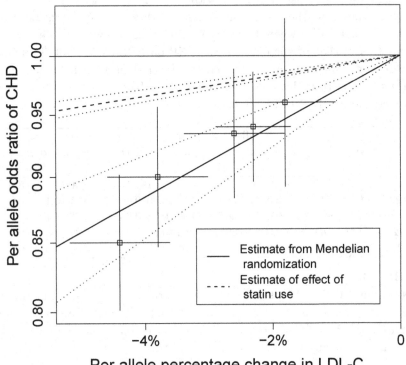

FIGURE 6.1

Estimates of percentage change in low-density lipoprotein cholesterol (LDL-C) and odds ratio of coronary heart disease (CHD) per LDL-C decreasing allele for five SNPs (point estimates with 95% confidence intervals), plus estimate of causal effect of LDL-C on CHD risk from Mendelian randomization using all five SNPs (solid line) with 95% confidence interval (dotted lines). Proportionate effect from meta-analysis of statin use on CHD risk in RCTs (dashed line with dotted lines for 95% confidence interval) is displayed for comparison.

The Mendelian randomization estimate of the effect of LDL-cholesterol reduction is greater (further from the null) than the estimate from RCTs of

LDL-cholesterol reduction using statins. It is known that the effect of statins in reducing CHD increases over time [Law et al., 2003]. As atherosclerosis is a chronic condition which develops progressively, it is not surprising that the estimates of the effect of the life-long lowering of LDL-cholesterol associated with the SNPs considered corresponds to a greater proportional change in cardiovascular risk than the effect on LDL-cholesterol due to statin usage. Further possible reasons for differences between the estimates include the non-specific action of statins, which also reduce inflammatory response [Davignon and Laaksonen, 1999]. However, any effects of statins on inflammatory response may further lessen the causal role of LDL-cholesterol, and make the contrast with the genetic effects more extreme.

6.2.2   Blood pressure and coronary heart disease

A similar example can be observed in the association between blood pressure and CHD. An allele score (Section 8.2) associated with a 1.6mmHg decrease in systolic blood pressure is associated with a odds ratio for CHD of 0.91 (95% CI 0.89 to 0.92) [Ehret et al., 2011]. Assuming a log-linear relationship, this corresponds to an odds ratio of 0.55 (95% CI 0.47 to 0.61) for a 10mmHg decrease in systolic blood pressure, compared to the relative risks from a meta-analysis of 0.78 (95% CI 0.73 to 0.83) in clinical trials and 0.75 (95% CI 0.73 to 0.77) in observational cohort studies [Law et al., 2009]. Again, the Mendelian randomization estimate of the effect of blood pressure lowering is greater (further from the null) than the estimates from both RCTs and observational studies.

6.3   Example: Lipoprotein(a) and coronary heart disease

Lipoprotein(a) is an assembly of a lipid, essentially a LDL particle, and a protein, known as apolipoprotein(a). From a genetic perspective, it is an unusual phenotype, as genetic variants in the *LPA* gene region explain over 60% of the variance in lipoprotein(a). The causal relationship between lipoprotein(a) and coronary heart disease (CHD) risk has been investigated in a number of Mendelian randomization investigations [Clarke et al., 2009; Kamstrup et al., 2009]. We here provide headline results from Burgess et al. [2018a], which aimed to predict the impact of a short-term reduction in lipoprotein(a) levels in order to inform trial design for a lipoprotein(a)-lowering agent.

Figure 6.2 shows 43 genetic variants in the *LPA* gene region that were all associated with lipoprotein(a) levels at a genome-wide level of significance ($p < 5 \times 10^{-8}$) in a multivariable regression analysis (conditional analysis). The associations plotted in the figure are the genetic associations from regression on each variant in turn in separate univariable regression analyses, and are all orientated to the minor (less common) allele. The genetic associations with lipoprotein(a) and with CHD risk appear approximately proportional, suggesting that the causal effect of lipoprotein(a) on CHD risk is log-linear, with the relative risk corresponding to a 50 mg/dL change in lipoprotein(a) around five times that of a 10 mg/dL change in lipoprotein(a). Addressing linearity in these genetic associations is only possible because of the existence of genetic variants that have considerable variation in their associations with the exposure, which is not the case for most risk factors.

Figure 6.3 shows estimates for LDL-cholesterol (left panel) and lipoprotein(a) (right panel). For LDL-cholesterol, we compare the genetic estimate from Mendelian randomization, the observational estimate from multivariable regression, and the estimate from short-term trials of statins. For lipoprotein(a), we compare the genetic estimate from Mendelian randomization and the observational estimate, and use the ratio between the genetic estimate and the trial estimate for LDL-cholesterol to predict the trial estimate for lipoprotein(a). This analysis makes the assumption that the ratio of the effect on CHD risk of life-long to short-term lowering is the same for LDL-cholesterol and for lipoprotein(a).

The fact that Mendelian randomization estimates are typically larger than estimates in trials has positive and negative implications. On the negative side, it means that estimates from Mendelian randomization investigations are likely to be overly optimistic. In this example, lipoprotein(a) would need to be lowered by around 100 mg/dL to have a similar risk reduction to that obtained from a 38 mg/dL (1 mmol/L) reduction in LDL-cholesterol. However, the clinical benefit is unlikely to be a 45% reduction in CHD risk as implied by the Mendelian randomization estimate, but instead a 22% reduction as implied by clinical trials of statins. On the positive side, it means that Mendelian randomization investigations are likely to have greater power to detect causal effects, and so null results from Mendelian randomization may be more convincing in implying that any benefit of a clinical intervention will at best be small.

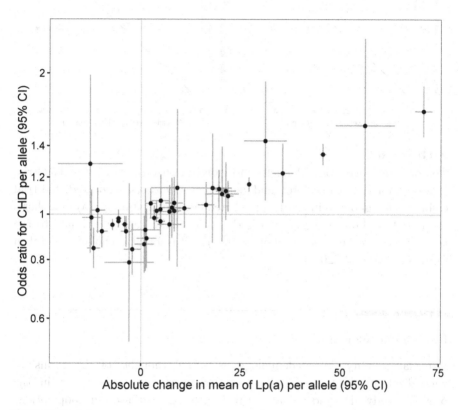

FIGURE 6.2

Genetic associations with lipoprotein(a) (horizontal axis, mg/dL) and with coronary heart disease (CHD) (vertical axis, odds ratios) for 43 genetic variants in the *LPA* gene region. Lines represent 95% confidence intervals for the genetic associations. Taken from Burgess et al. [2018a]. Some variants were only associated with lipoprotein(a) conditionally, and the confidence interval for the marginal association with lipoprotein(a) includes the null. Associations are orientated to the minor allele.

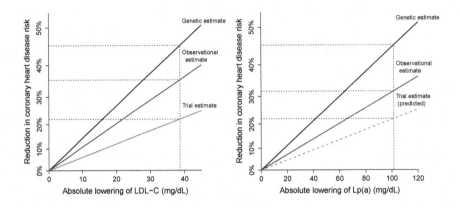

FIGURE 6.3

Comparison of genetic (Mendelian randomization), observational, and trial estimates for LDL-cholesterol, and genetic, observational, and predicted trial estimates for lipoprotein(a). The predicted effect of lipoprotein(a) in a short-term trial is obtained by assuming the ratio of the genetic estimate to the trial estimate is the same for lipoprotein(a) as it is for LDL-cholesterol. Taken from Burgess et al. [2018a].

6.4   Discussion

External validity in epidemiology is often thought of in terms of generalizability to a population other than the one considered in the original study [Dekkers et al., 2010]. Although variation in populations may cause some difficulties, the differences between the change in exposure levels associated with natural genetic variation and with any proposed clinical intervention on the exposure lead to inescapable problems in relating Mendelian randomization estimates to clinical questions of interest.

Mendelian randomization is a useful tool for exploring causal relationships between modifiable exposures and outcomes of interest. It is one of the few methodologies that can aid the selection of targets for therapeutic intervention. However, it would be misleading to assume that the estimate from a Mendelian randomization study gave the definitive answer to every question of causal relevance of an exposure. Mendelian randomization estimates are especially relevant when the effect of interest is that of a long-term population-based intervention; otherwise, although a Mendelian randomization approach may be qualitatively informative, the quantity estimated may not correspond to the clinical effect of interest.

6.4.1 Using Mendelian randomization in drug assessment

Questions of interpretation of results are important when using Mendelian randomization to prioritize or de-prioritize targets for drug development, especially in the context of the primary prevention of disease. A considerable proportion of large-scale and expensive clinical trials of drugs targeting suspected novel mechanisms of action fail to demonstrate efficacy. A prudent approach to drug development would be to prioritize targets where there is evidence on the causal nature of the exposure and/or mechanism from human genetics [Plenge et al., 2013]. Where suitable genetic variants for the application of Mendelian randomization on a given exposure are known and available in a large enough sample, assessment of the association between the variants and the disease outcome, and consequently of the causal effect of the exposure on the outcome, is simple, quick, and relatively inexpensive to perform.

Association between a relevant genetic variant affecting the exposure and the outcome may be taken as evidence for the potential efficacy of a drug affecting the exposure pathway. However, absence of evidence for such an association does not necessarily imply lack of efficacy. A drug which blocks a particular biological pathway may have a profound effect on downstream markers, which may lead to a substantially different effect on outcome compared to the slight changes associated with a genetic variant. Although we may expect Mendelian randomization in many circumstances to provide a good qualitative indication of the efficacy of clinical intervention, the magnitude of the Mendelian randomization estimate will not necessarily be a reliable guide to the potential benefit of a drug in practice. Additionally, in many cases the drug will be aimed at secondary disease prevention or targeted at a particular population group (such as individuals who have high or low levels of the exposure) rather than at the general population. As the randomization of genetic variants is valid only in the population, testing the genetic association with the disease in a sample population chosen according to their disease status or exposure value may lead to misleading inferences (ascertainment bias, Section 3.2.5).

The Mendelian randomization paradigm can also aid in target re-assessment (drug repositioning). If an existing drug has a genetic variant that mimics its effect, then an association of the variant with another outcome may indicate that the drug is also an effective treatment for that outcome. Equally, genetic associations can inform the assessment of mechanism-associated safety.

For example, a variant in the *GCKR* gene is associated with lower plasma glucose levels, but also with higher triglyceride levels [Beer et al., 2009]. This observation may suggest that additional monitoring of triglyceride levels would be advisable in clinical trials of glucokinase activators.

6.4.2   Using Mendelian randomization in drug discovery

'Reverse Mendelian randomization' can be used when a SNP is found in genome-wide association data to be associated with a disease outcome, but the mechanism for the association is not known. An exposure is sought which is associated with the variant and could explain the gene–disease association. This concept is closely related to that of functional genomics. For example, associations between variants in the *HMGCR* gene and risk of coronary heart disease are indicative of the causal role of low-density lipoprotein cholesterol in cardiovascular pathogenesis, and also point towards the potential efficacy of drugs to inhibit HMG-CoA reductase (statins). This approach should provide a fruitful source of targets for ongoing pharmacological research, and has already been used successfully in the discovery of the PCSK9 enzyme for cholesterol lowering (a variant in the *PCSK9* gene having been previously shown to be associated with CHD risk [Cohen et al., 2006]). PCSK9 inhibitors have now been demonstrated to be effective in lowering LDL-cholesterol [Robinson et al., 2014], and phase III trials have shown beneficial effects on cardiovascular endpoints.

6.4.3   Relevance of causal estimation in Mendelian
randomization

As has been emphasized throughout this book, Mendelian randomization investigations can assess a causal relationship, or estimate a causal effect. The arguments in this chapter suggest that the magnitude of causal effect estimates using Mendelian randomization should not be interpreted without critical thought. While they provide some indication of the potential relevance of an exposure, the direction of the causal effect and whether it is compatible or not with the null are more important.

Another reason for this is that the true causal risk factor may be difficult to define, and so the measured exposure may only be a surrogate (proxy) measure of the underlying risk factor. For example, in a Mendelian randomization analysis of the causal effect of BMI on disease, genetic variants associated with BMI may influence the outcome by causal pathways via other adiposity-related variables. In this case, formally the IV assumptions are violated as there is a causal pathway from the variants to the outcome not via the exposure

[Glymour et al., 2012]. However, if the investigation is interpreted not narrowly as estimating the causal effect of BMI on the outcome, but more broadly as estimating the causal effect of adiposity (for which BMI is used as a proxy measure) on the outcome, then the estimate may still a valid test of the causal null hypothesis if there is no causal pathway from the genetic variant(s) to the outcome not via adiposity, in spite of the IV assumptions for BMI being violated.

For these reasons, some authors have questioned whether causal effect estimates should ever be considered as part of a Mendelian randomization analysis [VanderWeele et al., 2014]. Although there is a danger of estimates being over-interpreted, there are several reasons why causal estimates are useful. First, in epidemiology generally, estimates with confidence intervals are preferred to hypothesis tests with p-values, as they are more informative [Sterne and Davey Smith, 2001]. For instance, if a p-value does not achieve conventional levels of statistical significance, a point estimate with a confidence interval allows the reader to judge in a quantitative way whether the null result reflects a lack of evidence or a genuine negative finding in comparison with either the observational association, or with a minimal clinically relevant effect. Secondly, if several genetic variants are valid instrumental variables for the same exposure, greater power to detect a clinically relevant causal effect can be obtained combining information on all of the variants into a single estimate rather than assessing the variant–outcome associations individually. Causal estimates from multiple variants also enable the quantitative comparison of the consistency of genetic associations, using a heterogeneity test, as a statistical assessment of pleiotropy (Section 5.3). Finally, although the causal estimate in a Mendelian randomization analysis may not be equal to the effect of the clinically-relevant intervention on the exposure, it does have a well-defined interpretation as an intervention on the genetic code at conception. Hence, although assessment of causation is typically be the primary outcome of a Mendelian randomization investigation, the estimate of a causal effect also has considerable utility.

6.5 Recap of examples considered so far

Before finishing the first part of the book, we pause to recall the examples of Mendelian randomization presented so far, remembering the statement in Chapter 2 that not all Mendelian randomization investigations are equal in terms of how they are performed or the strength of evidence they provide.

We have presented analyses for lipoprotein-associated phospholipase A_2 (Lp-PLA$_2$) using variants in the *PLA2G7* gene region (Section 3.4), and for interleukin-1 using variants in the *IL1RN* gene region (Section 5.1). In both cases, the risk factor was a protein (Lp-PLA$_2$ is an enzyme, interleukin-1 is a cytokine), and the gene region either encodes the protein (for Lp-PLA$_2$) or a closely-related protein (for interleukin-1, this was interleukin-1 receptor antagonist). Testing for a causal effect was the primary analysis of interest. The main justification for the instrumental variable assumptions is the specific link between the gene region and the exposure. The analysis of lipoprotein(a) using variants in the *LPA* gene region (Section 6.3) was similar, except in this case the causal estimate was also a key outcome from the analysis. We would argue with some confidence that causal inferences in these examples are reliable.

In contrast, we have presented analyses for LDL-cholesterol (Section 5.3 for Alzheimer's disease and Section 6.2.1 for CHD) and for BMI (Sections 4.3 and 5.5) using variants from multiple gene regions. For the analysis of LDL-cholesterol and CHD, we selected five variants in gene regions with known connection to LDL-cholesterol. The biological understanding of the gene regions and the consistency in the estimates between variants means that we are confident in the reliability of this analysis. For the analysis of LDL-cholesterol and Alzheimer's disease, we selected 75 genome-wide significant predictors of LDL-cholesterol. Once the two outliers were removed from the analysis, there was no residual evidence supporting a causal effect of LDL-cholesterol on Alzheimer's disease. Although it is unlikely that all the remaining variants are valid IVs, the absence of associations with Alzheimer's disease implies no evidence for a causal effect. While we could have restricted to a smaller set of genetic variants, a null finding including more variants can be considered more convincing: more variants means that power to detect a causal effect is greater, and no evidence supporting a causal effect was observed even including potentially pleiotropic variants in the analysis.

In the case of BMI, we selected up to 31 variants that were associated with BMI in a genome-wide association study, but otherwise we did not assess their relevance to BMI. In the analysis including 31 variants, evidence for a causal effect of BMI on cigarette smoking was observed. Here, no heterogeneity in the variant-specific causal estimates was observed in the analysis. This is reassuring, although further evidence justifying the IV assumptions would be welcome to strengthen the causal claim. Analyses for BMI were performed as a one-sample analysis using individual-level data, and as a two-sample analysis using summarized data; results were similar between these analyses. While performing similar analyses in two separate datasets can to some extent be considered a useful replication of the findings, if the IV assumptions are violated in one dataset, then they are also likely to be violated in the other dataset.

6.6 Summary

In Mendelian randomization, differences in the exposure distribution due to genetic variation are materially distinct from the change due to any proposed therapeutic intervention on the exposure, and so may affect the outcome differently. Consequently, it may be misleading to interpret the magnitude of a Mendelian randomization estimate as the expected impact of an intervention on the exposure in practice. Awareness of this is important for the use of Mendelian randomization in target-based drug development.

Part II

Advanced methods for Mendelian randomization

7

Robust methods using variants from multiple gene regions

In this part of the book, we describe more advanced methods for Mendelian randomization. We begin by considering robust methods, which do not require all genetic variants to be valid instrumental variables (IVs) to give consistent estimates of a causal parameter.

If a particular gene region (or regions) has a specific biological link to the exposure, then we would generally advocate basing the primary Mendelian randomization analysis on variants from that region. However, particularly for complex risk factors such as body mass index or blood pressure, there is no single gene region that encodes the risk factor, and so a polygenic Mendelian randomization analysis is necessary. If several genetic variants in different gene regions have similar associations with the outcome, then a polygenic analysis may even provide stronger evidence of a causal relationship, as the analysis is not dependent on the validity of the IV assumptions for a single gene region. However, in many cases, not all genetic variants associated with the exposure will tell the same story.

Three important factors when comparing methods are bias, coverage, and efficiency. Bias is the difference between the true value of a parameter and the average value of an estimate when it is calculated multiple times in independent datasets. If a method produces biased estimates, then on average the estimates from the method will be too large or too small compared to the true parameter value. Asymptotic bias means bias in the limiting case as the sample size increases towards infinity. Coverage is the probability that a confidence interval contains the true parameter value. By definition, a 95% confidence interval should contain the true parameter value 95% of the time. However, in practice, this may not be true, due to approximations and distributional assumptions made in constructing the interval. Coverage of a method under the null hypothesis is related to the Type 1 error rate (or false positive rate), in that if the coverage is $(1 - \alpha)$ then the Type 1 error rate is α. Maintaining a nominal Type 1 error rate (for instance, having a Type 1 error rate close to 5% for a test at a nominal 5% significance level) is especially important to avoid making false positive causal claims. Efficiency of an estimate relates to the power to detect a true causal effect. A method is more efficient if it produces estimates with smaller standard errors, and thus narrower confidence intervals and greater power.

7.1 Motivating example: LDL- and HDL-cholesterol and coronary heart disease

In Section 6.2.1, we showed that five genetic variants influencing low-density lipoprotein (LDL) cholesterol had associations with coronary heart disease (CHD) risk that were proportional to their associations with LDL-cholesterol. This is consistent with LDL-cholesterol being a causal risk factor for CHD, as has been demonstrated in randomized controlled trials. If rather than selecting variants with a specific biological link to LDL-cholesterol, we consider instead all 75 uncorrelated variants associated with LDL-cholesterol from a previous genome-wide association study (GWAS) [Do et al., 2013], then there is some additional heterogeneity in the genetic associations with the outcome, but a consistent story still emerges (Figure 7.1, left panel): the vast majority of genetic variants that are positively associated with LDL-cholesterol are also positively associated with CHD risk.

For high-density lipoprotein (HDL) cholesterol, the picture is different. We consider 86 uncorrelated genetic variants previously associated with HDL-cholesterol at a genome-wide level of significance, and display their associations with HDL-cholesterol and CHD risk in Figure 7.1 (right panel). We see that there is considerable heterogeneity in the variant-specific causal estimates, with some variants suggesting a positive causal effect of HDL-cholesterol on CHD risk, and others suggesting a negative causal effect. The inverse-variance weighted (IVW) method gives a log odds ratio of -0.160, corresponding to an odds ratio of 0.85 per 1 standard deviation increase in genetically-predicted HDL-cholesterol, with 95% confidence interval in a random-effects model from 0.76 to 0.95. However, Cochran's Q statistic is 439.7, corresponding to an I^2 statistic of 80.7%, suggesting that not all these genetic variants are valid IVs for HDL-cholesterol. Indeed, while trials of drugs that lower LDL-cholesterol have consistently shown reductions in CHD risk [Cholesterol Treatment Trialists' Collaboration, 2005; Sabatine et al., 2017], CETP inhibitors that raise HDL-cholesterol have generally shown null results in trials [Tardif et al., 2015; Lincoff et al., 2017].

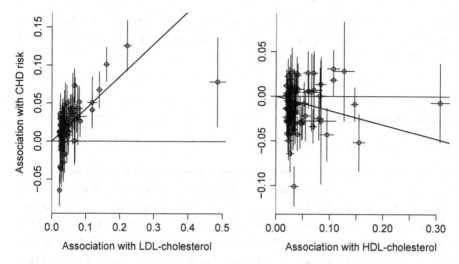

FIGURE 7.1

Genetic associations with LDL-cholesterol (left panel) and HDL-cholesterol (right panel, both standard deviation units) and with CHD risk (log odds ratios). Horizontal and vertical lines represent 95% confidence intervals for the genetic associations. Diagonal lines represent IVW estimates. Adapted from Burgess and Davey Smith [2017].

We consider robust methods for Mendelian randomization in three categories: consensus methods, outlier-robust methods, and modelling methods. Table 7.1 summarizes the methods presented.

As the majority of Mendelian randomization analyses are conducted using summarized data, we focus on methods that can be implemented using summarized data on genetic associations with the exposure ($\hat{\beta}_{Xj}$) and with the outcome ($\hat{\beta}_{Yj}$) and their standard errors (se($\hat{\beta}_{Xj}$) and se($\hat{\beta}_{Yj}$)), or else the variant-specific ratio estimates ($\hat{\theta}_j = \frac{\hat{\beta}_{Yj}}{\hat{\beta}_{Xj}}$) and their approximate standard errors (se($\hat{\theta}_j$) = $|\frac{\text{se}(\hat{\beta}_{Yj})}{\hat{\beta}_{Xj}}|$), for genetic variants $j = 1, \ldots, J$. We assume that all the variants are uncorrelated. While robust methods based on the IVW method can be adapted for correlated variants, it is likely that if one variant in a given gene region is an invalid IV, then other variants in the same gene region will also be invalid IVs. Hence if it is uncertain which variants are valid IVs, it is sensible to prune down to one genetic variant per gene region before proceeding with the analysis, to ensure that no gene region has a strong influence on the analysis. Throughout this chapter, we assume that all associations of the genetic variants with the exposure and outcome are homogeneous (that is, do not differ between individuals) and linear, and the effect of the exposure on the outcome is homogeneous and linear (Section 5.2.1).

7.2   Consensus methods

The two-stage least squares and inverse-variance weighted estimates can both be expressed as a weighted mean of the ratio estimates for the individual variants (Section 5.2.2). If the ratio estimates are close to zero for all but one of the genetic variants, but non-zero for just one variant, then the weighted mean of the ratio estimates will differ from zero. This implies that if the true causal effect is null, a single pleiotropic genetic variant can lead to rejection of the causal null hypothesis, a false positive finding. The property that a single incorrect datapoint can lead to an arbitrarily large bias in an estimate is referred to as a 0% breakdown point.

A consensus method is one that takes its causal estimate as a summary measure of the distribution of the variant-specific estimates. We consider the median method that has a 50% breakdown point ('majority valid' assumption) and the mode-based estimation method that has a higher breakdown point ('plurality valid' assumption).

7.2.1   Median method

The most straightforward consensus method is the median method [Bowden et al., 2016]. Rather than taking a weighted mean of the ratio estimates as in the IVW method, we take the median of the ratio estimates. Under the linearity and homogeneity assumptions of Section 5.2.1, all genetic variants that are valid instrumental variables estimate the same causal parameter. In a large sample size, this means that the ratio estimates for the valid IVs will all tend towards the same value. Provided that over 50% of the genetic variants are valid IVs, this means that the median of the ratio estimates will tend towards the true causal effect. In a finite sample size, estimates from invalid IVs will still influence the median estimate, but they will have far less influence than for the IVW estimate (Figure 7.2).

In the simple median method, all genetic variants receive equal weight in the analysis. A weighted version of the median method can also be calculated. In the weighted median method, we consider an empirical distribution in which each variant receives a weight corresponding to the inverse of the variance of

Method	Consistency assumption	Strengths and weaknesses	Reference
Inverse-variance weighted	All valid or balanced pleiotropy	Most efficient (greatest statistical power), biased if average pleiotropic effect differs from zero	Burgess et al. [2013]
Weighted median	Majority valid	Robust to outliers, sensitive to addition/removal of genetic variants	Bowden et al. [2016]
Mode-based estimation	Plurality valid	Robust to outliers, sensitive to bandwidth parameter and addition/removal of genetic variants, often less efficient	Hartwig et al. [2017]
MR-PRESSO	Outlier-robust	Removes outliers, efficient with valid IVs, very high false positive rate with several invalid IVs	Verbanck et al. [2018]
MR-Robust	Outlier-robust	Downweights outliers, efficient with valid IVs, high false positive rate with several invalid IVs	Rees et al. [2019b]
MR-Lasso	Outlier-robust	Removes outliers, efficient with valid IVs, high false positive rate with several invalid IVs	Rees et al. [2019b]
MR-Egger	InSIDE	Robust to pleiotropy under InSIDE assumption, sensitive to outliers, sensitive to violations of InSIDE assumption, InSIDE assumption often not plausible, often less efficient	Bowden et al. [2015]
Contamination mixture	Plurality valid	Robust to outliers, sensitive to variance parameter and addition/removal of genetic variants	Burgess et al. [2020b]
MR-Mix	Plurality valid	Robust to outliers, requires large numbers of genetic variants, very high false positive rate in several scenarios	Qi and Chatterjee [2019b]
MR-RAPS	Balanced pleiotropy (except outliers)	Downweights outliers, sensitive to violations of balanced pleiotropy assumption	Zhao et al. [2018]

TABLE 7.1

Comparison of robust methods. This list is not exhaustive, but focuses on methods that can be implemented using summarized genetic associations. InSIDE = instrument strength independent of direct effect (see Section 7.4.1).

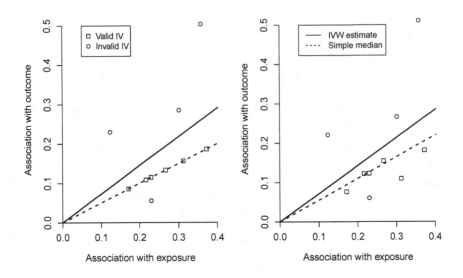

FIGURE 7.2

Illustration of simple median method: synthetic data on genetic associations with exposure and outcome corresponding to infinite sample size (left panel) and finite sample size (right panel) for six valid instruments (squares) and four invalid instruments (circles). Solid lines represent IVW estimates, dashed lines represent simple median estimates.

the ratio estimate (the same weights as in the IVW method). Estimates are ranked in order, and the weighted median estimate is taken as the estimate at the median (the 50th percentile) of the empirical distribution.

For example, suppose there are five variants, and the variant with the lowest estimate receives 25% of the weight, the next variant 20%, the third variant 15%, the fourth variant 30%, and the variant with the largest estimate 10%. The 50th percentile of the empirical distribution is between the estimates for the second and third variants. As the cumulative weight at the second variant is 45% and the cumulative weight at the third variant is 60%, we extrapolate linearly taking the second estimate plus $\frac{50-45}{60-45} = \frac{5}{15} = \frac{1}{3}$ of the difference between the third and second estimates. This is equivalent to taking two-thirds of the second estimate plus one-third of the third estimate.

Standard errors and confidence intervals for the median method are constructed by parametric bootstrapping of the genetic association estimates, making a normal assumption for the estimate. We refer to the assumption that over 50% of the variants are valid IVs as the 'majority valid' assumption.

For the weighted median method, it is required that over 50% of the weight corresponds to valid IVs.

7.2.2 Mode-based estimation method

Suppose that there is an even number of genetic variants and, as the sample size increases, exactly half of them have ratio estimates that tend to one value, and the other half tend to a different value. Under the majority valid assumption, we would not be able to tell which group of variants represents the valid IVs, and which represents the invalid IVs. However, suppose instead that 40% of the variants tend towards one value, 10% towards a second value, 10% towards a third value, 10% towards a fourth value, and so on. These values cannot all be the true causal effect of the exposure on the outcome. We may reasonably state that there is more weight of evidence that the value evidenced by the 40% of variants is the true causal effect. The 'plurality valid' assumption states that out of all the different values taken by ratio estimates in large samples (we term these the ratio estimands), the true causal effect is the value taken for the largest number of genetic variants (that is, the modal ratio estimand) [Guo et al., 2018]. This assumption allows the true causal effect to be identified in cases where less than 50% of variants are valid IVs, provided that no larger group of invalid IVs with the same ratio estimand exists. This assumption is also referred to as the Zero Modal Pleiotropy Assumption (ZEMPA) [Hartwig et al., 2017].

This assumption is exploited by the mode-based estimation method [Hartwig et al., 2017]. As no two ratio estimates will be identical in finite samples, it is not possible to take the mode of the ratio estimates directly. In the mode-based estimation method, a normal density is constructed for each genetic variant centered at its ratio estimate. The spread of this density depends on a bandwidth parameter, and (for the weighted version of the mode-based estimation method) the precision of the ratio estimate. A smoothed density function is then obtained by summing these normal densities. The maximum of this distribution is the causal estimate. Again, confidence intervals are constructed by parametric bootstrapping with a normal assumption on the distribution of the causal estimate.

7.2.3 Summary of consensus methods

As these consensus methods take the median or mode of the ratio estimate distribution as the causal estimate, they are naturally robust to outliers, as the median and mode of a distribution are unaffected by the magnitude of extreme values. However, they are still influenced by invalid variants, as these variants contribute to determining the location of the median or mode of a distribution. These methods can also be particularly sensitive to changes in the ratio estimates for variants that contribute to the median or mode, and to the addition and removal of variants from the analysis. Additionally, the methods may not be as efficient as those that combine the estimates from multiple genetic variants more directly. In particular, the mode-based method has been shown to be less efficient than other methods [Slob and Burgess, 2020].

7.3 Outlier-robust methods

Next, we present three outlier-robust methods. These methods either downweight or remove genetic variants from the analysis that have outlying ratio estimates. They provide consistent estimates under the same assumptions as the IVW method for the set of genetic variants that are not identified as outliers.

7.3.1 MR-PRESSO method

In the MR-Pleiotropy Residual Sum and Outlier (MR-PRESSO) method [Verbanck et al., 2018], the IVW method is implemented by weighted regression using all the genetic variants, and the residual sum of squares (RSS) is calculated from the regression equation. The RSS is a measure of heterogeneity, and is equal to Cochran's Q statistic. Then, the IVW method is performed omitting each genetic variant from the analysis in turn. If the RSS decreases substantially compared to a simulated expected distribution, then that variant is removed from the analysis. This procedure is repeated until no further variants are removed from the analysis. The causal estimate is then obtained by the IVW method using the remaining genetic variants.

7.3.2 MR-Robust method

In MR-Robust, the IVW method is again implemented by weighted linear regression, except that instead of using least squares regression, MM-estimation is used combined with Tukey's biweight loss function [Rees et al., 2019b]. MM-estimation (each 'M' stands for 'maximum likelihood type') provides robustness against influential points and Tukey's loss function provides robustness against outliers. Tukey's loss function is a truncated quadratic function, meaning that there is a limit in the extent to which an outlier contributes to the analysis [Mosteller and Tukey, 1977]. This contrasts with the quadratic loss function used in least squares regression, which is unbounded, meaning that a single outlier can have an unlimited effect on the IVW estimate.

7.3.3   MR-Lasso method

In MR-Lasso, the IVW regression model is augmented by adding an intercept term for each genetic variant [Rees et al., 2019b]. From the weighted regression model in equation (5.6), the IVW estimate is the value of θ that minimizes:

$$\sum_{j=1}^{J} \text{se}(\hat{\beta}_{Yj})^{-2} \left(\hat{\beta}_{Yj} - \theta\, \hat{\beta}_{Xj} \right)^2. \tag{7.1}$$

In MR-Lasso, we minimize:

$$\sum_{j=1}^{J} \text{se}(\hat{\beta}_{Yj})^{-2} \left(\hat{\beta}_{Yj} - \theta_{0j} - \theta\, \hat{\beta}_{Xj} \right)^2 + \lambda \sum_{j=1}^{J} |\theta_{0j}|, \tag{7.2}$$

where λ is a tuning parameter. As the regression equation contains more parameters than there are genetic variants, a lasso penalty term is added for identification [Windmeijer et al., 2018]. The intercept term θ_{0j} represents the direct (pleiotropic) effect of the jth variant on the outcome. It should be zero for a valid IV, but will be non-zero for an invalid IV. The causal estimate is then obtained by the IVW method using the genetic variants that had $\hat{\theta}_{0j} = 0$ in equation (7.2). A heterogeneity criterion is used to determine the value of λ. Increasing λ means that more of the pleiotropy parameters equal zero and so the corresponding variants are included in the analysis; we increase λ step-by-step until one step before there is more heterogeneity in the ratio estimates for variants included in the analysis than expected by chance alone.

The MR-Lasso method is a summarized data version of the Some Invalid Some Valid Instrumental Variables Estimator (sisVIVE) method [Kang et al., 2016]. The sisVIVE method proposes a similar model relating the IVs, exposure, and outcome, but expressed in terms of individual-level data.

7.3.4   Summary of outlier-robust methods

The MR-PRESSO and MR-Lasso methods remove variants from the analysis, whereas MR-Robust downweights variants. These methods will be valuable when there is a small number of genetic variants with heterogeneous ratio estimates, as they will be removed from the analysis or heavily downweighted, and so will not influence the overall estimate. In such a case, these methods are likely to be efficient, as they are based on the IVW method. The methods are likely to be less valuable when there is a larger number of genetic variants that are mildly pleiotropic, or when the average pleiotropic effect of non-outliers is not zero.

One note of caution: if these methods remove a substantial proportion of the variants from the analysis, they may give a false impression of confidence in the causal estimate due to homogeneity of the ratio estimates amongst the remaining variants. However, it is not reasonable to claim that there is strong evidence for a causal effect after a large number of variants with heterogeneous estimates have been removed from the analysis.

7.4   Modelling methods

Finally, we present four robust methods that attempt to model the distribution of estimates from invalid IVs or make a specific assumption about the way in which the IV assumptions are violated.

7.4.1   Decomposition of genetic associations and the IVW method

Before introducing the remaining robust methods, we consider a parametric decomposition of the genetic associations with the outcome. We write the association of the jth variant as:

$$\beta_{Yj} = \alpha_j + \theta\,\beta_{Xj} \tag{7.3}$$

where α_j is the pleiotropic (direct) effect of the genetic variant on the outcome, and $\theta\,\beta_{Xj}$ is the causal (indirect) effect of the genetic variant on the outcome via the exposure, which comprises the genetic association with the exposure (β_{Xj}) multiplied by the causal effect of the exposure on the outcome (θ). Note that these quantities are written without hats, indicating that the decomposition is for the parameters, rather than their estimates.

The ratio estimand (that is, the quantity targeted by the ratio estimate) for the jth variant can therefore be written as:

$$\frac{\beta_{Yj}}{\beta_{Xj}} = \frac{\alpha_j + \theta\,\beta_{Xj}}{\beta_{Xj}} = \theta + \frac{\alpha_j}{\beta_{Xj}}. \tag{7.4}$$

This is equal to the causal effect θ if and only if $\alpha_j = 0$, which occurs when the pleiotropic effect of the variant is zero. It can be similarly shown that the IVW estimand is equal to θ when a weighted average of the pleiotropic effects of the variants is zero and a weighted correlation between the α_j and the β_{Xj} is zero [Burgess et al., 2016a]. This condition is referred to as 'balanced pleiotropy'. The IVW method therefore provides a consistent estimate of the causal effect either under the assumption that all variants are valid IVs ('all valid') or the assumption of balanced pleiotropy.

The condition that the weighted correlation between the α_j and the β_{Xj} is zero is referred to as the 'InSIDE' assumption – I̲nstrument S̲trength I̲ndependent of D̲irect E̲ffect.

7.4.2   MR-Egger method

The MR-Egger method [Bowden et al., 2015] is performed similarly to the IVW method, except that the regression model contains an intercept term θ_0:

$$\hat{\beta}_{Yj} = \theta_0 + \theta\,\hat{\beta}_{Xj} + \varepsilon_j, \quad \varepsilon_j \sim \mathcal{N}(0, \text{se}(\hat{\beta}_{Yj})^2). \tag{7.5}$$

The estimate of the slope parameter θ is the MR-Egger estimate. This method differs from the MR-Lasso method, as there is only one intercept term θ_0, which represents the average pleiotropic effect. The MR-Egger method gives consistent estimates of the causal effect under the InSIDE assumption. In contrast to the IVW method, the average pleiotropic effect does not have to be equal to zero, and (under the InSIDE assumption) will be estimated by the intercept term θ_0. The average pleiotropic effect not equalling zero is referred to as 'directional pleiotropy'.

The intercept in MR-Egger also provides a test of the IV assumptions. The intercept will differ from zero when either the average pleiotropic effect is not zero, or the InSIDE assumption is violated. These two conditions (average pleiotropy of zero and InSIDE assumption satisfied) are precisely those required for the IVW estimate to be unbiased (balanced pleiotropy).

An intuitive way of thinking about the MR-Egger method is that it assesses whether there is a dose–response relationship between the genetic associations with the exposure and those with the outcome. Illustrative data are shown in Figure 7.3. For the synthetic data in the left panel, although all five of the genetic variants individually suggest a positive causal effect of the exposure on the outcome, a dose–response relationship in the associations is absent. Genetic variants that have a greater magnitude of association with the exposure do not also have a greater magnitude of association with the outcome. This is contrary to what would be expected if the associations of the genetic variants with the outcome were entirely mediated via the exposure, and hence it is unlikely that all of the genetic variants are valid instrumental variables. While the individual ratio estimates are all positive (as is the IVW estimate), the MR-Egger regression model (dashed line) tells a different story. The intercept term from MR-Egger differs from zero, and the causal estimate from MR-Egger is compatible with the null. This suggests that the set of genetic variants suffers from directional pleiotropy and, once this pleiotropy is accounted for, there is no residual evidence for a causal effect.

A similar conclusion applies to the example of plasma urate and CHD risk in Figure 7.3 (right panel). Estimates (odds ratio per 1 standard deviation increase in genetically-predicted plasma urate with 95% confidence interval) are 1.11 (1.03, 1.20) for the IVW method, and 1.00 (0.90, 1.10) for the MR-Egger method [Burgess and Thompson, 2017].

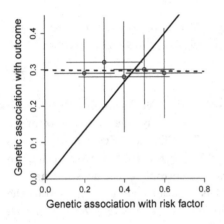
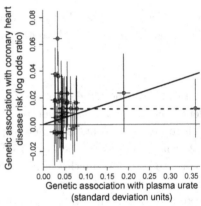

FIGURE 7.3
Graph showing genetic associations for synthetic (left panel) and real data (right panel) examples in which inverse-variance weighted estimate (solid line) and MR-Egger estimate (dashed line) differ substantially. Horizontal and vertical lines are 95% confidence intervals for the genetic associations. In both cases, the inverse-variance weighted estimate is positive, whereas the MR-Egger causal estimate is null with intercept term differing from zero. Taken from Burgess and Thompson [2017].

As the MR-Egger regression model is not invariant to changes in the signs of the genetic association estimates (which would result from switching the reference and effect alleles), we first re-orientate the genetic associations before performing the MR-Egger method by fixing all genetic associations with the exposure to be positive, and correspondingly changing the signs of the genetic associations with the outcome if necessary.

7.4.3   Difficulties with the MR-Egger method

Readers who are familiar with robust methods for Mendelian randomization may be surprised that MR-Egger is not the first robust method presented in this chapter, despite being the first such method to be developed. While the method can be useful, there are several potential issues with its use.

First, while the re-orientation of genetic associations is necessary to ensure that estimates from the MR-Egger method do not depend on an arbitrary choice of effect alleles, the dependence of the method on a specific orientation of the genetic associations is not ideal. Changing the orientation of a variant affects the definition of the pleiotropic effect α_j. There are therefore different versions of the InSIDE assumption for each of the potential choices of orientation of the variants, and it is only possible for these all to be satisfied if all the pleiotropic effects are zero.

Secondly, the precision of the MR-Egger estimate is not dependent on the proportion of variance in the exposure explained by the genetic variants (as for the IVW method), but on the variance between the genetic associations with the exposure. If these associations are all similar (as in Figure 7.4, left panel), then the MR-Egger estimate will have wide confidence intervals. The precision of the MR-Egger estimate will always be less than that of the IVW estimate, and the difference in precision can be substantial.

Thirdly, the MR-Egger estimate can be strongly influenced by individual variants. In Figure 7.4 (left and right panels), we see how the addition of a single genetic variant can reverse the sign of the MR-Egger estimate, and lead to rejection of the MR-Egger intercept test. The influence on the IVW estimate is less severe.

Finally, the InSIDE assumption is generally implausible when variants are pleiotropic [Burgess and Thompson, 2017]. If the pleiotropic effects of genetic variants act via confounders, then the InSIDE assumption will typically be violated even if they influence the outcome via different confounders. If variants influence the outcome via the same confounder, then violation will be more severe still. Even if the pleiotropic effects are not via confounders, for any particular set of genetic variants the correlation between pleiotropic effects and genetic associations with the exposure is likely to differ from zero, meaning that the InSIDE assumption is violated and the MR-Egger estimate is biased.

In favour of MR-Egger, the InSIDE assumption is very different to the majority or plurality valid and outlier-robust assumptions. Robust methods that make the majority or plurality assumption, and so rely on several genetic variants being valid IVs, are likely to give similar answers. In contrast, the MR-Egger method allows all genetic variants to be invalid IVs. However, instead,

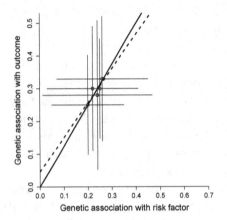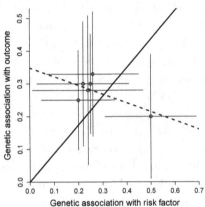

FIGURE 7.4

Synthetic data on genetic associations of five genetic variants (left panel) and with the addition of one extra variant (right panel). Left panel: IVW estimate (solid line) and MR-Egger estimate (dashed line) are similar. Right panel: IVW estimate (solid line) and MR-Egger estimate (dashed line) are markedly different, and the influential genetic variant changes the sign of the MR-Egger estimate. Taken from Burgess and Thompson [2017].

it relies on the variants satisfying the InSIDE assumption, an untestable and perhaps still implausibly strong assumption.

7.4.4 Contamination mixture method

The contamination mixture method assumes that only some of the genetic variants are valid IVs, and provides consistent estimates under the plurality valid assumption [Burgess et al., 2020b]. To perform the method, a likelihood function is constructed from the ratio estimates. If a variant is a valid instrument, then its ratio estimate $\hat{\theta}_j$ is assumed to be normally distributed about the true causal effect θ with variance $\text{se}(\hat{\theta}_j)^2$. If a variant is not a valid instrument, then its ratio estimate is assumed to be normally distributed about zero with variance $\psi^2 + \text{se}(\hat{\theta}_j)^2$, where ψ^2 represents the variance of the estimands from invalid IVs. This parameter is specified by the analyst. We then maximize the likelihood over different values of the causal effect θ and different configurations of valid and invalid IVs. Maximization is performed by first constructing a profile likelihood as a function of θ, and then maximizing this function with respect to θ. The value of θ that maximizes the profile likelihood is the causal estimate. Confidence intervals are constructed using the likelihood function, and do not rely on bootstrapping or normality of the parameter estimate. The confidence interval is typically not symmetric, and is not even guaranteed to be a single range of values. A confidence interval comprising multiple disjoint ranges occurs when there is uncertainty which of two or more groups of variants supporting different causal effects has more weight of evidence.

7.4.5 MR-Mix method

The MR-Mix method [Qi and Chatterjee, 2019b] is similar to the contamination mixture method, except that rather than dividing the genetic variants into valid and invalid IVs, the method divides variants into four categories: 1) variants that directly influence the exposure only (valid IVs), and 2) variants that influence the exposure and outcome, 3) variants that influence the outcome only, and 4) variants that influence neither the exposure nor outcome. This allows for more flexibility in modelling genetic variants, although potentially leads to more uncertainty in assigning genetic variants to categories.

7.4.6   MR-RAPS method

The MR-Robust Adjusted Profile Score (RAPS) [Zhao et al., 2018] method models the pleiotropic effects of genetic variants directly using a random-effects distribution. The pleiotropic effects are assumed to be normally distributed about zero with unknown variance, independently of the genetic associations with the exposure. Estimates are obtained using a profile likelihood function for the causal effect and the variance of the pleiotropic effects distribution. To provide further robustness to outliers, either Tukey's biweight loss function or Huber's loss function [Mosteller and Tukey, 1977] can be used.

7.4.7   Summary of modelling methods

Modelling methods are likely to be valuable when the modelling assumptions are correct, but not when the assumptions are incorrect. For example, the MR-Egger method requires the InSIDE assumption to be satisfied to give a consistent estimate. The MR-RAPS method is likely to perform well when pleiotropic effects are truly normally distributed about zero, but less well when they are not. The MR-Mix method is likely to require large numbers of genetic variants in order to correctly classify variants into the different categories. The contamination mixture method is less likely to be affected by modelling assumptions as it does not make such strict assumptions, but it can be sensitive to specification of the variance parameter.

7.5   Other methods and comparison

As stated at the beginning of the chapter, we have focused on robust methods that can be implemented using summarized data. Another method that satisfies this criterion fits a similar model to the MR-Lasso method with one pleiotropic parameter per variant, except instead of using lasso penalization to identify the pleiotropic effects of the different variants, it takes a Bayesian approach and imposes a prior distribution on the pleiotropic effects [Berzuini et al., 2020]. Other methods that require individual-level data include: the MR GENIUS method (G-Estimation under No Interaction with Unmeasured Selection), which exploits orthogonality conditions to allow for arbitrary additive pleiotropy functions [Tchetgen Tchetgen et al., 2017]; a constrained optimization approach that includes data on genetic associations with potential confounders, attempting to maximize the association of a linear combination of genetic variants with the exposure while minimizing associations with the confounders [Jiang et al., 2019]; and a confidence interval method that aims to identify groups of variants having similar causal estimates [Windmeijer et al., 2019].

Comparison of different robust methods is difficult. While methods can be compared as to their theoretical properties, it is often unclear how relevant these properties are in practice. The value of comparisons based on simulated data is unclear, as each method typically performs well when its assumptions are satisfied, and poorly when they are not. Comparisons based on real data are difficult to interpret, as there are few examples of exposure–outcome pairs where we are confident to state that the exposure is a causal risk factor for the outcome. Two comparisons of robust methods are Slob and Burgess [2020] and Qi and Chatterjee [2019a]: these investigations prioritized the contamination mixture method and the MR-Mix method as having the best estimation properties. However, these methods were each developed by the authors of the respective comparisons. We discuss recommendations for practice in Section 10.6: in brief, we recommend comparing results from a range of methods that make different assumptions. For example, investigators could perform the weighted median, MR-Egger, and contamination mixture methods. Alternatively, the contamination mixture method could be replaced by the mode-based estimation method or the MR-Mix method.

7.6 Example: LDL- and HDL-cholesterol and coronary heart disease reprised

We return to the examples of LDL- and HDL-cholesterol and risk of CHD using genome-wide significant variants introduced at the beginning of the chapter. We proceed to perform the IVW method and each of the robust methods presented in this chapter in turn. Default options were used for each method, including random-effects models and weights for the mode-based estimation method. We recall that clinical trials suggest that LDL-cholesterol is a causal risk factor for CHD, but suggest that HDL-cholesterol may not be.

Results are given in Table 7.2. For LDL-cholesterol, estimates from all methods are positive and the 95% confidence intervals all exclude the null. For HDL-cholesterol, estimates are more variable. Estimates from the weighted median, mode-based estimation, and MR-Egger methods are attenuated towards the null, and the 95% confidence intervals include the null. The MR-Egger intercept excludes the null, suggesting violation of the InSIDE

assumption and/or directional pleiotropy. The confidence interval from the
contamination mixture method consists of two disjoint ranges, suggesting
that there are two groups of variants supporting different effect estimates
(see Burgess et al. [2020b] for a discussion of this). Estimates from the
outlier-robust methods are all similar, and the confidence intervals from these
methods exclude the null.

While we would discourage comparing methods based on their results for a
single dataset, for HDL-cholesterol we see disagreement between the estimates
from different methods, indicating that there is less confidence in a causal
finding for HDL-cholesterol compared with for LDL-cholesterol.

Method	LDL-cholesterol Estimate (95% CI)	HDL-cholesterol Estimate (95% CI)
IVW	1.530 (1.402, 1.669)	0.852 (0.764, 0.951)
Simple median	1.525 (1.389, 1.675)	0.767 (0.679, 0.867)
Weighted median	1.587 (1.454, 1.732)	0.953 (0.867, 1.048)
Mode-based estimation	1.699 (1.509, 1.912)	0.993 (0.903, 1.092)
MR-PRESSO	1.530 (1.402, 1.669)	0.852 (0.764, 0.951)
MR-Robust	1.610 (1.448, 1.791)	0.864 (0.764, 0.976)
MR-Lasso	1.615 (1.528, 1.707)	0.861 (0.803, 0.923)
MR-Egger	1.605 (1.391, 1.852)	1.102 (0.930, 1.306)
(intercept)	-0.003 $(-0.011, 0.005)$	-0.015 $(-0.023, -0.007)$
Contamination mixture	1.679 (1.597, 1.783)	0.671 (0.595, 0.772 and 0.888, 0.953)
MR-Mix	1.716 (1.587, 1.856)	0.549 (0.409, 0.736)
MR-RAPS	1.570 (1.457, 1.692)	0.879 (0.797, 0.970)

TABLE 7.2

Comparison of estimates from different robust methods for the effect of LDL-
and HDL-cholesterol on CHD risk. Estimates represent odds ratios (95%
confidence intervals) per 1 standard deviation increase in genetically-predicted
values of the lipid fraction, except for the MR-Egger intercept, which is the
untransformed regression coefficient.

7.7 Computer implementation

Several robust methods are implemented for R in the *MendelianRandomization* package available from the Comprehensive R Archive Network (CRAN) [Yavorska and Burgess, 2017]. The median method is implemented as:

```
mr_median(mr_input(bx, bxse, by, byse), weighting="simple")
mr_median(mr_input(bx, bxse, by, byse), weighting="weighted")
```

The mode-based method is implemented as:

```
mr_mbe(mr_input(bx, bxse, by, byse))
```

The MR-Robust method is implemented as:

```
mr_ivw(mr_input(bx, bxse, by, byse), robust=TRUE)
```

The MR-Lasso method is implemented as:

```
mr_lasso(mr_input(bx, bxse, by, byse))
```

The MR-Egger method is implemented as:

```
mr_egger(mr_input(bx, bxse, by, byse))
```

The contamination mixture method is implemented as:

```
mr_conmix(mr_input(bx, bxse, by, byse))
```

The MR-PRESSO method is implemented using the *MR-PRESSO* package, available from `https://github.com/rondolab/MR-PRESSO`. The MR-Mix method is implemented using the *MRMix* package, available from `https://github.com/gqi/MRMix`. The MR-RAPS method is implemented using the *mr.raps* package, available from the CRAN.

The median, mode-based, and MR-Egger methods are implemented for Stata in the *mrrobust* package [Spiller et al., 2019].

7.8 Summary

In this chapter, we have presented a wide range of robust methods for Mendelian randomization. Findings from a polygenic Mendelian randomization investigation are more reliable when several methods that make different assumptions give similar answers. However, each of these methods still relies on untestable assumptions, and appropriate caution in their interpretation is needed, particularly when results from methods differ.

8

Other statistical issues for Mendelian randomization

In this chapter, we discuss various statistical issues affecting estimates from Mendelian randomization. While it is not possible to completely separate theoretical and pragmatic considerations, the focus of this chapter is more on understanding why and how these methodological issues affect findings. Practical advice on how to perform Mendelian randomization investigations in the light of these issues is presented in Chapter 10.

In turn, we discuss weak instrument bias, allele scores, sample overlap, winner's curse, selection and collider bias, covariate adjustment, non-collapsibility, time and time-varying effects, power, choosing variants from a single gene region, binary exposures, and alternative estimation methods. As in the previous chapter, we particularly focus on factors affecting the bias, coverage, and efficiency of estimates.

While there is a logical order in which the issues are presented, readers may wish to focus on those sections most relevant to their interest. Further information on these issues is available in the references provided.

8.1 Weak instrument bias

A weak instrument is an instrumental variable (IV) that is not strongly associated with the exposure in statistical terms [Burgess and Thompson, 2011]. A weak instrument is still a valid IV, in that it satisfies the IV assumptions. Estimates based on a weak instrument are asymptotically unbiased (that is, the bias decreases to zero as the sample size increases towards infinity). But for any finite sample size, estimates will be biased.

8.1.1 Explanations of weak instrument bias

A valid instrument will be distributed independently of all confounders, meaning that in a theoretical infinite sample size, the correlation between the instrument and confounders will be exactly zero. However, in a finite sample the correlation will not be exactly equal to zero.

For simplicity of explanation, we consider the case in which the IV takes two values (0 and 1) and there is a single confounding variable [Nelson and Startz, 1990]. The average difference in the outcome between the genetic subgroups comprises two components, a systematic component owing to the effect of the genetic variant on the exposure, and a random component owing to the association of the genetic variant with the confounder. There will also be a further component owing to chance differences that do not relate to the confounder, but we assume this component is negligible. If the genetic variant is a strong instrument, then the average difference in the outcome between genetic subgroups will be mainly due to the genetic effect on the exposure. However if the instrument is weak, the chance difference in the confounder will account for proportionally more of the difference.

We can demonstrate the effect of this chance difference algebraically. We first consider a one-sample setting, and assume the continuous exposure X can be expressed as a linear function of the genetic variant G and the confounder U, and the continuous outcome Y can be expressed as a linear function of the exposure and confounder as follows:

$$X = \alpha_0 + \alpha_1 G + \alpha_2 U + \varepsilon_X \tag{8.1}$$
$$Y = \theta_0 + \theta_1 X + \theta_2 U + \varepsilon_Y.$$

Now, the average difference in the exposure between the two genetic subgroups is $\Delta X = \alpha_1 + \alpha_2 \Delta U + \Delta \varepsilon_X$, and the average difference in the outcome between the two genetic subgroups is $\Delta Y = \theta_1 \Delta X + \theta_2 \Delta U + \Delta \varepsilon_Y$, where ΔU is the average difference in the confounder between the two subgroups, and $\Delta \varepsilon_X$ and $\Delta \varepsilon_Y$ are the average differences in the error terms between the two subgroups. If $\Delta \varepsilon_X$ and $\Delta \varepsilon_Y$ are exactly zero, the ratio IV estimate is:

$$\frac{\Delta Y}{\Delta X} = \frac{\theta_1 \Delta X + \theta_2 \Delta U}{\Delta X} = \theta_1 + \frac{\theta_2 \Delta U}{\alpha_1 + \alpha_2 \Delta U}. \tag{8.2}$$

When ΔU is exactly zero, the second term disappears and the IV estimate is equal to θ_1, the true causal effect of the exposure on the outcome. If α_1, which represents the effect of the genetic variant on the exposure, is large compared with $\alpha_2 \Delta U$, then the denominator of the second term will be large compared with the numerator, and again the IV estimate will be close to θ_1. However, as α_1 tends towards zero, then the IV estimate tends to $\theta_1 + \frac{\theta_2}{\alpha_2}$, where the second term is calculated from the effects of the confounder on the outcome and exposure. Hence, as the effect of the genetic variant on the exposure gets closer to zero, then the bias of the IV estimate approaches the association between exposure and outcome resulting from changes in the confounders, which is the bias of the observational confounded association [Bound et al., 1995].

In a two-sample setting, the average difference in the confounder in sample one will be independent of the average difference in the confounder in sample two. Hence rather than the ΔU terms in the ratio IV estimate cancelling, the ΔU in the numerator will be different from the ΔU in the denominator.

Bias can also be explained with reference to results from the measurement error literature [Willett, 1989]. In the two-stage least squares (2SLS) method, if the IVs are weak then the fitted values of the exposure from the first-stage regression will be estimated with uncertainty. In a two-sample setting, this is equivalent to non-differential measurement error. The coefficient for the fitted values of the exposure in the second-stage regression, which is the causal estimate, is attenuated to the null. In a one-sample setting, random errors in the exposure and outcome are correlated, and bias is in the direction of the correlation between the two error terms, which is due to confounding.

A final explanation of weak instrument bias is illustrated in Figure 8.1. This represents the output from 1000 synthetic datasets simulated for a scenario in a one-sample setting in which there is a strong positive correlation between the exposure and outcome due to confounding, but a negative causal effect of the exposure on the outcome [Burgess and Thompson, 2011]. We assume there is a genetic variant that divides the population into three equal-sized subgroups. Each point on the figure represents the mean level of the exposure and outcome in a genetic subgroup of the population for one of the simulated datasets. The plotting symbol and shade of points relates to the subgroup of the population; all points representing the same subgroup are presented in the same shade of grey. Differences between the subgroup estimates are due to the systematic effect of the genetic variant on the exposure. Differences within the subgroup estimates are, at least in part, due to differences in the chance correlation of the genetic variant with the confounder.

To examine the sampling distribution of the IV estimate, we take one point at random from each of the three subgroup distributions, and draw the regression line for these points. The gradient of the line is the IV estimate. When the instrument is strong (top-left panel), the large differences in the exposure between the subgroups will generally lead to a negative estimate of the effect of the exposure on the outcome. When the instrument is weak (bottom-right panel), the differences in exposure between the subgroups due to the IV are small and the positively confounded observational association is more likely to be recovered. In a two-sample setting, the subgroup distributions would be horizontally-flattened ellipses in shape rather than skewed in the direction of the confounded association, leading to flattening of the gradient and hence bias towards the null.

8.1.2   Causal estimates with weak instruments

As stated above, in a one-sample setting, bias due to weak instruments is in the direction of the observational association between the exposure and outcome. The magnitude of the bias depends on the expected value of the F statistic from regression of the exposure on the IVs. The relative bias of the IV estimate from the 2SLS method, defined as the bias of IV estimate divided by the bias of the observational estimate, is approximately equal to $1/\mathbb{E}(F)$, where $\mathbb{E}(F)$ is the expected value of the F statistic [Staiger and Stock, 1997]. This approximation is only valid when the number of IVs is at least three.

The F statistic is related to the proportion of variance in the exposure explained by the genetic variants (R^2), sample size (N) and number of instruments (K) by the formula $F = (\frac{N-K-1}{K})(\frac{R^2}{1-R^2})$. For a single variant, the F statistic is equal to the square of the genetic association with the exposure divided by the square of its standard deviation:

$$\text{F statistic} = \left(\frac{\hat{\beta}_X}{\text{se}(\hat{\beta}_X)}\right)^2 \tag{8.3}$$

Alternatively, for a biallelic SNP, R^2 can be approximated as $2\,\beta_X^2\,MAF\,(1-MAF)$ where β_X is the genetic association with the exposure measured in standard deviation units of the exposure, and MAF is the minor allele frequency. As an example, a biallelic SNP associated with a 0.15 standard deviation increase in the exposure per additional allele and a minor allele frequency of 30% would explain $2 \times 0.15^2 \times 0.3 \times 0.7 = 0.009 = 0.9\%$ of the variance in the exposure. For uncorrelated genetic variants, the total proportion of variance explained can be summed across variants. For correlated variants, the proportion explained can be calculated using the Cholesky decomposition of the inverse of the correlation matrix for the genetic variants.[1]

An often cited rule-of-thumb is that an F statistic less than 10 indicates the presence of weak instruments. This derives from the observation that when $\mathbb{E}(F) < 10$, the bias of the IV estimate is more than 10% of the bias in

---

[1]In R syntax, the proportion is: `sum(2*(beta_x%*%solve(chol(rho)))^2*maf*(1-maf))` where `beta_x` is the vector of genetic associations in standard deviation units, `rho` is the matrix of correlations between genetic variants, and `maf` is the vector of minor allele frequencies.

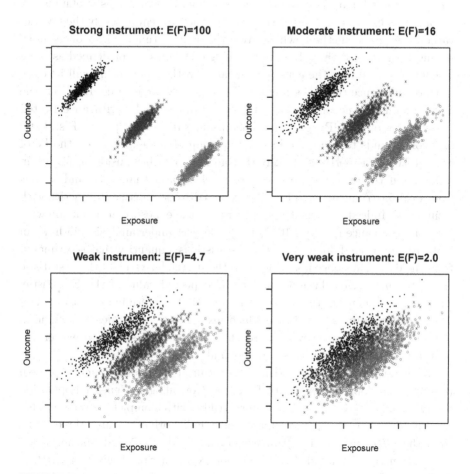

FIGURE 8.1

Distribution of mean outcome and mean exposure levels in three genetic subgroups (indicated by different symbols and shades of grey) for various strengths of the instrument, with expected values of the F statistic (see Section 8.1.2). One point of each colour comes from each of the 1000 simulated datasets. The IV estimate for each simulated dataset is the gradient of the regression line for the three points.

the observational association estimate (relative bias $> 1/10$). However, there are many caveats to the use of this rule in practice. First, the rule gives the impression that an IV is either weak or not weak, whereas in reality instrument strength is not binary and there is no threshold at which bias is eliminated. Second, this bias only relates to the 2SLS method (or equivalently the inverse-variance weighted method, which gives the same estimate) in a one-sample setting with at least three IVs. With a single IV, bias is not defined as there is a small chance that the genetic association with the exposure will be close to zero, and hence the IV estimate will take a very large value. However, the median value of the bias is close to zero even for an IV with an expected F statistic around 5 [Burgess and Thompson, 2011]. An expected F statistic of 5 corresponds to a p-value in the regression of the exposure on the IV of around 0.03. It is perhaps unlikely that an IV would be considered for use in a dataset if the expected p-value were much greater than 0.03, and so bias from weak instruments would not be expected to be an issue in practice with a single IV. Indeed, a variant associated with the exposure at a genome-wide level of significance ($p < 5 \times 10^{-8}$) in the dataset under analysis will have an F statistic of around 30. Finally, the F statistic is a quantity that is estimated from the data. Bias does not depend on the particular value of the F statistic calculated in a given dataset, but on the expected value of the F statistic. This means that using the observed F statistic to determine how to analyse the data (for example, to choose which instruments or studies to include in the analysis) is a data-driven approach, and has been shown to exacerbate bias rather than to lessen bias [Burgess and Thompson, 2011].

To demonstrate this, we estimate the causal effect of C-reactive protein (CRP) on fibrinogen using data from the Copenhagen General Population Study [Zacho et al., 2008], a cohort study with complete cross-sectional baseline data for 35 679 participants on CRP, fibrinogen, and three SNPs from the *CRP* gene region [Burgess et al., 2011]. CRP and fibrinogen are observationally correlated, but we do not expect a causal effect of CRP on fibrinogen. We calculate the observational estimate by regressing fibrinogen on log(CRP), and the IV estimate by the 2SLS method using all three SNPs as IVs in a per allele additive model (Section 4.2.1). We then analyse the same data as if it came from multiple smaller studies by dividing the data randomly into substudies of equal size, calculating estimates of association in each substudy, and combining the results using inverse-variance weighted fixed-effect meta-analysis. We divide the whole study into, in turn, 5, 10, 16, 40, 100, and 250 substudies.

We see from Table 8.1 that the observational estimate stays almost unchanged whether the data are analysed as one study or as several studies. However, as the number of substudies increases, the pooled IV estimate increases from near zero until it approaches the observational estimate. At the same time, the standard error of the pooled IV estimate decreases. We can see that even where the number of substudies is 16 and the average F statistic is around 10, there is a serious bias. The causal estimate with 16 substudies is positive ($p = 0.09$) despite the causal estimate with the data analysed as one study being near to zero.

Substudies	Observational estimate	2SLS IV estimate	Mean F statistic
1	1.68 (0.01)	−0.05 (0.15)	152.0
5	1.68 (0.01)	−0.01 (0.15)	31.4
10	1.68 (0.01)	0.09 (0.14)	16.4
16	1.68 (0.01)	0.23 (0.14)	10.8
40	1.68 (0.01)	0.46 (0.13)	4.8
100	1.67 (0.01)	0.83 (0.11)	2.5
250	1.67 (0.01)	1.27 (0.08)	1.6

TABLE 8.1

Estimates of effect (standard error) of log(CRP) on fibrinogen (μmol/l) from the Copenhagen General Population Study ($N = 35\,679$) divided randomly into substudies of equal size and combined using fixed-effect meta-analysis: observational estimates using unadjusted linear regression, IV estimates using 2SLS. Mean F statistics from linear regression of log(CRP) on three genetic variants are averaged across substudies.

Figure 8.2 shows the estimates from these 16 substudies using the 2SLS method with their corresponding F statistics. The substudies which have greater estimates are the ones with larger F statistics; the correlation between F statistics and point estimates is 0.83. The substudies with higher F statistics also have tighter confidence intervals and so receive more weight in the meta-analysis. This is the opposite result to what may have been anticipated, as we said above that larger expected F statistics result in less bias. However, in this artificial example, the expected value of the F statistic is the same in all substudies, and so the IVs are truly no stronger in the substudies with $F > 10$ than in those with $F < 10$.

If we exclude from the meta-analysis substudies with an F statistic less than 10, then the pooled estimate increases from 0.23 (SE 0.14, $p = 0.09$) to 0.43 (SE 0.16, $p = 0.006$). Equally, if we only use as instruments in each substudy the IVs with an F statistic greater than 10 in a univariate regression on the exposure, then the pooled estimate increases to 0.28 (SE 0.15, $p = 0.06$). So neither of these approaches are useful in reducing bias.

Although the expectation of the F statistic is a good indicator of bias, the observed F statistic shows considerable variation. In the 16 substudies

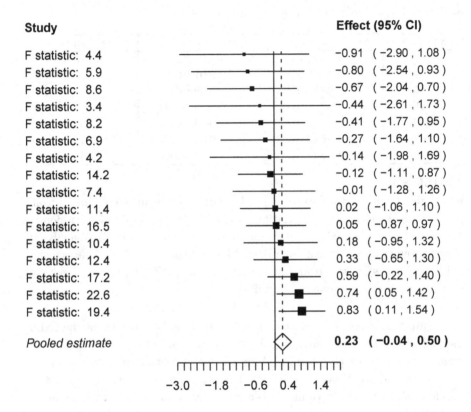

FIGURE 8.2
Forest plot of causal estimates of log(CRP) on fibrinogen (μmol/l) using data from the Copenhagen General Population Study divided randomly into 16 equally sized substudies (each $N \simeq 2230$). Studies are ordered by their causal estimate. F statistics are calculated from regression of the exposure on the three IVs. Size of markers is proportional to the weight assigned to the substudy in a fixed-effect meta-analysis.

of Figure 8.2, the measured F statistic ranges from 3.4 to 22.6. In more realistic examples, all other factors being equal, studies with higher expected F statistics would tend to also have higher observed F statistics, and hence have truly stronger instruments and less bias. However, the sampling variation of causal effects and observed F statistics in each study would still tend to follow the pattern of Figure 8.2, with overestimated F statistics corresponding to more biased causal estimates. So while it is desirable to use strong instruments, the measured strength of instruments in the data under analysis is not a good guide to the true instrument strength.

8.1.3 Inferences with weak instruments

In addition to problems of bias, IV estimates with weak instruments can have underestimated coverage [Stock and Yogo, 2002; Mikusheva and Poi, 2006]. Confidence intervals from Fieller's theorem (Section 4.1.5), which are not constrained to be symmetric (or even finite), result in better coverage properties. Alternatively, confidence intervals from inverting a test statistic, such as the Anderson–Rubin test statistic [Anderson and Rubin, 1949] or the conditional likelihood ratio test statistic [Moreira, 2003] give appropriate confidence levels under the null hypothesis with weak instruments [Mikusheva, 2010]. These can be implemented using the *ivmodel* software package in R [Kang et al., 2020].

In a one-sample setting, bias under the null hypothesis leads to inflated Type 1 error rates. In a two-sample setting, there is no bias under the null hypothesis, as any bias would be towards the null, which is the true causal effect [Pierce and Burgess, 2013]. Hence IV estimates in a two-sample setting do not suffer from inflated Type 1 error rates. Even in a one-sample setting, testing the association between the outcome and each IV in turn (without estimating a causal effect) provides valid tests of a causal relationship even with weak instruments.

A further problem with weak instruments is instrument invalidity. If two invalid IVs have pleiotropic effects of the same size, then the IV estimate from the weaker IV will be more biased [Small and Rosenbaum, 2008]. For a weak instrument, even a slight association with a confounder can lead to severe bias. Although all methods for Mendelian randomization are influenced by weak instruments, the MR-Egger method is particularly susceptible to bias, and is not recommended for use in a one-sample setting with weak instruments [Hartwig and Davies, 2016].

8.1.4   Reducing bias from weak instruments

As the bias in 2SLS IV estimates depends on the expected F statistic in the regression of the exposure on the IV, bias can be reduced by increasing the expected F statistic [Burgess et al., 2011]. The F statistic depends on the sample size, so bias can be reduced by increasing the sample size. Similarly, if there are instruments that are not explaining much of the variation in the exposure, then excluding these instruments will increase the F statistic. In general, employing fewer parameters to model the genetic association will increase the F statistic. Ideally, issues of weak instrument bias should be addressed prior to data collection, by specifying sample sizes, instruments, and genetic models using the best prior evidence available to ensure that the expected value of the F statistic is large.

8.2   Allele scores

An allele score (also called a genetic risk score, gene score, or genotype score) is a single variable summarizing multiple genetic variants in a univariate score [Burgess and Thompson, 2013], and is a popular approach used in Mendelian randomization. An unweighted allele score is constructed as the total number of exposure-increasing alleles present in the genotype of an individual. A weighted allele score can also be considered, where each allele contributes a weight reflecting the effect of the corresponding genetic variant on the exposure. These weights can be derived internally from the data under analysis, or externally from an independent data source.

If an individual i has g_{ij} copies of the exposure-increasing allele for each variant $j = 1, \ldots, J$, then their unweighted score is $\sum_{j=1}^{J} g_{ij}$. This score takes integer values between 0 and $2J$. If the weight for variant j is w_j, then their weighted score is $\sum_{j=1}^{J} w_j g_{ij}$.

There are two main reasons for using an allele score. The first is parsimony. As an example, the validity of the IV assumptions can be explored by testing the association of each variant with a set of measured covariates. However, when the numbers of variants and covariate traits are large, this may be impractical. Instead, the association of the allele score with the covariates can be tested. Assessment of IV violations with a single score variable will be simpler to present, and power to detect a violation will be improved if several variants have pleiotropic associations with the same covariate.

The second reason is to reduce weak instrument bias. As noted above, median bias with a single IV is close to zero even for relatively weak IVs.

Hence, combining multiple genetic variants into an allele score is a potential strategy for reducing weak instrument bias. If the allele score is weighted using genetic associations with the exposure from the dataset under analysis, then the weighted allele score is mathematically equivalent (up to an additive constant) to the fitted value of the exposure used in the 2SLS method. In this case, the ratio IV estimate using the allele score is the same as the 2SLS estimate, and weak instrument bias is not avoided. If weights are derived from the dataset under analysis, it would be misleading to present an F statistic for the allele score as if it is a single variable. However, if the allele score is weighted using genetic associations with the exposure from a second dataset, then this is equivalent to a two-sample analysis. In this case, weak instrument bias is towards the null and does not result in inflated Type 1 error rates.

While use of an unweighted allele score seems like a crude approach, it can be used to reduce weak instrument bias if a second dataset to estimate the weights is not available. Although there is some loss of power associated with using an unweighted rather than a weighted score, this loss is not large if the genetic variants have fairly similar magnitudes of association with the exposure. A related loss of power is suffered in using a weighted score approach if the weights are imprecisely estimated [Burgess and Thompson, 2013].

Alternatively, weights can instead be estimated using the data under analysis in a cross-validation approach, by dividing the data into equal sized parts, and constructing an allele score using weights in each part estimated using the data from all the other parts [Burgess and Thompson, 2013]. For example, in a two-fold cross-validation analysis, genetic associations with the exposure are estimated in one half of the data. These are used as weights to construct an allele score and then estimate associations of the score with the exposure and outcome in the other half of the data. Then, genetic associations with the exposure are estimated in the second half of the data and used to construct an allele score. Associations of the score with the exposure and outcome are then estimated in the first half of the data. The two resulting IV estimates are then combined using meta-analysis. A more sophisticated approach is a 10-fold cross-validation, in which 10 sets of weights are estimated. Weights used for constructing the allele score in each tenth of the sample are obtained from the remaining 90% of the sample. As the weights are estimated using more of the data, estimates should be more precise.

The use of an allele score in Mendelian randomization requires the assumption that the allele score is an instrumental variable. This means that each variant which contributes to the allele score must satisfy the assumptions of an instrumental variable. The only exception to this is the first assumption: while the inclusion of a genetic variant that is not associated with the exposure will not improve the score, it will not make the score an invalid IV.

A disadvantage of using an allele score is that it eliminates the possibility of assessing heterogeneity in the variant-specific causal estimates; using an allele score is similar to performing a fixed-effect meta-analysis (Section 5.3.1).

8.3   Sample overlap

While the two-sample setting leads to reduced severity of weak instrument bias, this is generally a fortuitous side-effect rather than a deliberate strategic choice. The motivation for a two-sample analysis is often pragmatic: genetic associations with the exposure are available in one dataset, and genetic associations with the outcome in another dataset. However, due to the nature of major international genetics consortia, often the datasets are not completely disjoint, and some studies and participants are in common between the two datasets (Figure 8.3). When there is some overlap, it is unclear whether bias due to weak instruments would be in the direction of the null (as in the case of zero overlap) or in the direction of the observational association (as in the case of complete overlap) [Burgess et al., 2016b].

Bias in the 2SLS method depends on the covariance of the error terms in the first and second stages [Nagar, 1959]. This means that bias depends on the degree of sample overlap in a linear way. With summarized data, bias depends on the covariance between the variant–exposure and variant–outcome associations. Covariance is reduced if either the number of those in the variant–exposure dataset is low as a proportion of those in the variant–outcome dataset, or the number of those in the variant–outcome dataset is low as a proportion of those in the variant–exposure dataset. For example, if the smaller dataset has 1000 participants, and the larger dataset has 10 000 participants, then the sample overlap is only 10% even if all of the participants from the smaller dataset are included in the larger dataset. This is the case whether the smaller dataset is for the genetic associations with the exposure or with the outcome. In both cases, with 10% sample overlap, bias of the IV estimate in the direction of the observational association would be 10% of what would be observed with 100% sample overlap. An online tool for estimating bias and Type 1 error inflation due to sample overlap is available at https://sb452.shinyapps.io/overlap/.

One notable case is with a binary outcome. Provided that only control participants are used in estimation of the variant–exposure associations (Section 4.1.4), sample overlap will not lead to bias in the direction of the observational association even in a one-sample setting, as the variant–exposure

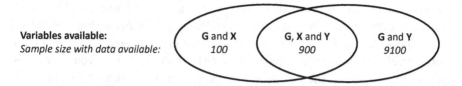

Variables available:	G and X	G, X and Y	G and Y
Sample size with data available:	*100*	*900*	*9100*

FIGURE 8.3

Schematic diagram for illustrative example on sample overlap showing the sample size with data available on G and X (left), G and Y (right), and G, X and Y (central intersection), where G indicates the genetic variants, X the exposure, and Y the outcome. The sample overlap in this example is 9%, as sample overlap is expressed with respect to the larger dataset, and out of the 10 000 individuals with data on G and Y, only 900 also have data on X.

and variant–outcome association estimates will be uncorrelated. Any weak instrument bias will follow the pattern of a two-sample setting [Burgess et al., 2016b]. However, if both controls and cases are used to estimate the variant–exposure associations, weak instrument bias will follow the pattern of a one-sample setting.

8.4 Winner's curse

Another bias occurs if the genetic variants used in a Mendelian randomization analysis were initially discovered in the data under analysis. This is due to a phenomenon known as winner's curse. If several genetic variants in truth have similar magnitudes of association with the exposure, the association of the one that is the strongest in the data under analysis is likely to be overestimated [Taylor et al., 2014]. As overestimation will generally occur when the associations with confounders are by chance stronger than expected, bias will arise if the discovery dataset is used in the estimation of the variant–exposure or the variant–outcome associations. Overlap between the discovery dataset and the dataset for the variant–outcome associations is a particular cause for concern, as this would result in overestimation of the variant–outcome associations and could lead to false positive findings.

Often a pragmatic decision has to be made as to what data to include in a Mendelian randomization analysis. It would be ideal if data on three large non-overlapping datasets were available from the same underlying population to ensure that genetic discovery, variant–exposure, and variant–outcome associations were estimated in independent samples. However, if this is not possible, or if restricting to non-overlapping datasets would lead to a substantial decrease in the sample size for the analysis, then a compromise is necessary to balance the risk of severe bias against the risk of an imprecise estimate and hence an uninformative finding.

8.5 Selection and collider bias

Selection bias and collider bias can influence findings from any analysis of observational data [Cole et al., 2010]. A collider is a common effect of two variables. An example of collider bias is illustrated in Figure 8.4.

In Mendelian randomization, the exposure is influenced by the genetic variants and any exposure–outcome confounders, and so is a collider on the causal pathway from the genetic variants to the outcome. Any downstream consequence of a collider is itself also a collider. If two variables are unrelated

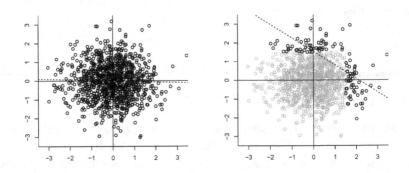

FIGURE 8.4

Diagram illustrating collider bias for synthetic data on two variables drawn from independent standard normal distributions. For the full dataset (left panel), correlation between the two variables (indicated by the dashed line) is close to zero. If we select by restricting to observations for which the maximum of the two variables is greater than 1.5 (right panel, points in black), then a strong negative correlation between the two variables is observed (dashed line). Collider bias occurs as this maximum is a function of the two variables, and hence is a collider for these variables on a causal diagram.

(they are marginally independent), they will typically be related when conditioning on the collider (they become conditionally dependent).

Stratifying on or adjusting for the exposure or any downstream consequence of the exposure (including the outcome) therefore leads to an association between the genetic variants and the exposure–outcome confounders in the strata. Such an association would lead to biased causal estimates.

Selection bias is a specific example of collider bias which occurs when selection into a study sample depends on a collider [Hernán et al., 2004]. Selection bias could occur when considering a secondary disease outcome, such as disease progression or a recurrent disease event. In order to be included in an analysis of disease progression, a participant must have had an initial disease event. If the exposure is a risk factor for the initial disease event, then selection into the sample population would be a function of a collider (namely, the exposure), and hence bias would occur. Secondly, selection bias could occur when considering genetic associations with a disease outcome in an elderly population, as a participant can only contribute to such an analysis if they have survived to old age (also known as survivor bias). Thirdly, selection bias could occur when considering causal effects in a subset of the population. For example, a large meta-analysis considered associations of genetic variants related to alcohol consumption with oesophageal cancer separately in non-drinkers, moderate drinkers, and heavy drinkers (Figure 8.5). Stronger associations were observed in heavier drinkers [Lewis and Davey Smith, 2005]. Selection bias would have occurred here, as strata were defined by the exposure. In contrast, sex-stratified analyses of alcohol-related variants should not be affected by selection bias, as sex is not a collider variable (it is determined at conception, and so cannot be an effect of any other variable) [Cho et al., 2015].

However, in the alcohol example of Lewis and Davey Smith [2005], differences observed between genetic associations with the outcome in non-drinkers, moderate drinkers, and heavy drinkers were implausibly large to be explained solely by collider bias. Simulation studies have shown that selection bias can have a severe impact on Mendelian randomization estimates, but only when the effect of the collider on selection is strong [Gkatzionis and Burgess, 2019; Hughes et al., 2019]. Selection bias can potentially be addressed using inverse-probability weighting, although this requires estimation of the probability of selection into the study sample for all individuals in the population [Gkatzionis and Burgess, 2019].

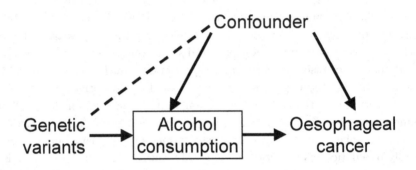

FIGURE 8.5
Directed acyclic graph of IV assumptions for the example of Lewis and
Davey Smith [2005] evaluating the causal effect of alcohol consumption on risk
of oesophageal cancer. By stratifying on alcohol consumption, the association
between the genetic variants and oesophageal cancer is estimated conditional
on alcohol consumption, which is the exposure. As the exposure is a common
effect of the genetic variants and confounders (a collider), conditioning on the
exposure induces a correlation between the genetic variants and confounders
indicated by the dashed line. The magnitude of this correlation depends on the
strength of the effects of the genetic variants and confounders on the exposure.
Although the effect of confounders on the exposure is not known, a sensitivity
analysis can be performed for this parameter to obtain the likely magnitude
of the collider bias. This allows the investigator to judge whether any genetic
association with the outcome can be explained solely by collider bias.

8.6   Covariate adjustment

In a classical observational analysis, it is necessary to adjust for a wide variety of confounding variables to plausibly argue that any association of the exposure with the outcome is due to a causal effect of the exposure (and even still, we would be sceptical of such a claim). In contrast, in a randomized controlled trial, it is not necessary to adjust for any covariates to obtain valid causal inferences. Nonetheless, there are two motivations for adjusting for covariates in a randomized trial: to improve efficiency and to reduce bias arising from chance covariate imbalance between the randomized subgroups [Steyerberg et al., 2000]. In an IV analysis, adjustment for covariates is similarly not necessary, but may improve efficiency and reduce chance covariate imbalance, which in an IV analysis leads to weak instrument bias. Covariate adjustment can be performed in the 2SLS method by including covariates in the first- and second-stage regression models, and in the inverse-variance weighted method by including covariates in the estimation of the variant–exposure and variant–outcome regression coefficients.

However, there are also potential pitfalls of including covariates in a Mendelian randomization analysis. Adjustment would bias estimates either if the covariate is on the causal pathway from the genetic variants to the outcome (a mediator), or if adjustment induces collider bias. In general, we would only recommend including as covariates: age, sex, genomic principal components of ancestry, and technical covariates (such as recruitment centre), unless there is strong justification otherwise. Adjustment for genomic principal components of ancestry is performed to mitigate against bias due to population stratification (Section 3.2.5) [Price et al., 2006]. Age and sex cannot be colliders or mediators on a causal pathway, as they are not caused by any variable in the model, so adjustment for these variables should improve precision of estimates without risking bias. Ideally, the same covariates should be adjusted for in both stages for the 2SLS method (with individual-level data) or both in the variant–exposure and variant–outcome associations for the inverse-variance weighted method (with summarized data) [Angrist and Pischke, 2009b]. However, practical considerations may make this difficult, particularly when using publicly-available summarized data, where the choice of covariate adjustment has already been made.

8.7   Non-collapsibility

Some measures of effect, including odds ratios, differ depending on whether they are considered conditional or marginal on a covariate. The left half of Table 8.2 provides illustrative data in which the odds ratio of an outcome for exposed versus unexposed individuals is equal to 2 for men and 2 for women. Even with no confounding (that is, the proportion of exposed and non-exposed individuals is the same in both men and women), the odds ratio for a population with equal numbers of men and women is not 2. In contrast, as the example in the right half of Table 8.2 shows, the relative risk is the same whether considered conditional or marginal on sex.

	Probability of event		Odds	Probability of event		Relative
	Unexposed	Exposed	ratio	Unexposed	Exposed	risk
Men	$\frac{3}{13}$	$\frac{3}{8}$	2	0.3	0.6	2
Women	$\frac{1}{21}$	$\frac{1}{11}$	2	0.05	0.1	2
Overall	0.139	0.233	1.88	0.175	0.35	2

TABLE 8.2
Illustrative examples of collapsing an effect estimate over a covariate: non-equality of conditional and marginal odds ratios and equality of relative risks. Analyses in men and women are conditional analyses (conditional on sex), whereas the overall analysis is marginal on sex.

A measure of effect, such as an odds ratio or relative risk, is collapsible in a covariate if, when it is constant across the strata of the covariate, this constant value equals the value obtained from the overall (marginal) analysis. Non-collapsibility is the violation of this property [Greenland et al., 1999]. The relative risk and absolute risk difference are collapsible measures of association. Odds ratios are in general non-collapsible [Ducharme and LePage, 1986].

An odds ratio estimated in a classical observational study by conventional multivariable logistic regression is conditional on those covariates adjusted for in the analysis. Unless adjustment is made in the IV analysis, an odds ratio estimated in a Mendelian randomization study is marginal on these covariates. The odds ratio from a two-stage or inverse-variance weighted method with no covariate adjustment is conditional on the IV, but marginal in all other variables [Burgess and CCGC, 2013]. This provides another reason why estimates from Mendelian randomization analyses may differ to those from other study designs (see also Chapter 6). However, an IV analysis with a binary outcome does still target a meaningful parameter, which represents the population-averaged change in the outcome for a shift in the distribution of the exposure [Burgess and Thompson, 2012]. It also provides a valid test of the null hypothesis since, if a measure of effect is zero in each of the strata, then it is zero when averaged across the strata [Vansteelandt et al., 2011]. Unless the binary outcome is common, bias due to non-collapsibility of the odds ratio in practice is generally not substantial [Burgess, 2017].

8.8   Time and time-varying effects

There is typically a large gap between the time when an individual's genotype is determined (at conception) and when the exposure and outcome are measured. Hence, Mendelian randomization investigations are generally not well-placed to address detailed questions about the timings of causal effects. In general, Mendelian randomization can only find evidence relating to the causal null hypothesis that no intervention on the exposure at any point in time affects the outcome [Swanson et al., 2018].

Mendelian randomization estimates relate specifically to changes in the exposure induced by the genetic variants used as IVs. The genetic code is fixed at conception, and so Mendelian randomization investigations typically compare groups of the population having different trajectories in their distribution of the exposure over time [Swanson et al., 2017]. Analyses therefore typically can be interpreted as assessing the impact of long-term elevated levels of an exposure. However, in most cases, we have incomplete information about how the genetic variant changes the distribution of the exposure across the life course. If the genetic associations with the exposure vary over time, then Mendelian randomization estimates based on genetic associations with the exposure measured at a single timepoint can be unreliable [Labrecque and Swanson, 2019].

Similar difficulties of interpretation arise if the impact on the outcome relates to levels of the exposure at a specific time period in life. A plausible example of this is the effect of vitamin D on multiple sclerosis; multiple sclerosis risk is hypothesized to be influenced by vitamin D levels during early childhood, but not vitamin D levels in adulthood [Holmes et al., 2017]. An assessment of whether there is a critical period at which the exposure influences the outcome would require comparison of genetic variants that influence the exposure to a different extent at different points in the life course. This may be possible for an exposure such as BMI, as different genetic variants are associated with BMI in adolescence, young adulthood, and older adulthood [Richardson et al., 2020]. A similar analysis has been performed for blood pressure, showing that midlife blood pressure influences coronary heart disease risk independently of later life blood pressure [Gill et al., 2020].

8.8.1   Time-to-event data

While we have discussed continuous outcomes and binary outcomes, we have so far omitted discussion of survival outcomes that are typically measured in a longitudinal study. Classical observational analyses of survival outcomes often estimate hazard ratios in a multiplicative hazard model using Cox proportional hazards regression. However, the causal interpretation of a hazard ratio is unclear [Hernán, 2010]. The hazard ratio at a particular timepoint is defined with respect to a risk set, which is the group of individuals who have been followed up until that time and have not yet experienced the event of interest. Conditioning on membership of a risk set is problematic, as this induces collider bias when the exposure is a causal risk factor for survival. An alternative proposal is to assume an additive hazard model and estimate a hazard difference [Martinussen et al., 2017]. This is a viable alternative, and a two-stage method using Aalen additive hazards regression has been proposed to perform IV analysis [Tchetgen Tchetgen et al., 2015]. However, there are several practical reasons why proportional hazards models are generally preferred to additive hazards models. For instance, the hazard function in an additive hazards model is not guaranteed to be always positive for all individuals in the population [Burgess, 2015]. Additionally, the causal effect of the exposure, whether estimated in an additive or multiplicative model, must be assumed to be constant in time.

Two pragmatic suggestions are either to proceed with estimating a hazard ratio or hazard difference (depending on whether a multiplicative or additive effect of the exposure is more plausible), but to interpret the estimate as a test statistic for the causal null hypothesis rather than a meaningful causal parameter, or to ignore the time-to-event outcome and analyse the data as a binary outcome. The first approach is still a valid test of the causal null hypothesis [Tchetgen Tchetgen et al., 2015], and can be implemented using a two-stage method (with Cox proportional hazards or Aalen additive hazards regression in the second-stage model) or the inverse-variance weighted method (with summarized genetic associations as beta-coefficients from proportional or additive hazards regression). The second approach ignores censoring and differences in event times between individuals, and so will be less efficient when individuals have been followed up over a long period.

8.9 Power to detect a causal effect

With a single IV and a continuous outcome, the asymptotic variance of the IV estimate $\hat{\theta}_{IV}$ from the ratio or 2SLS method is:

$$\text{var}(\hat{\theta}_{IV}) = \frac{\text{var}(R_Y^{IV})}{N \, \text{var}(X) \, \rho_{GX}^2} \tag{8.4}$$

where N is the sample size, $R_Y^{IV} = Y - \hat{\theta}_1 X$ is the residual of the outcome after subtraction of the estimated causal effect of the exposure, and ρ_{GX}^2 is the square of the correlation between the exposure X and the IV G. The coefficient of determination (R^2) in the regression of the exposure on the IV is an estimate of ρ_{GX}^2.

The asymptotic variance of the conventional regression (ordinary least squares, OLS) estimate $\hat{\beta}_{OLS}$ is:

$$\text{var}(\hat{\theta}_{OLS}) = \frac{\text{var}(R_Y^{OLS})}{N \, \text{var}(X)} \tag{8.5}$$

where $R_Y^{OLS} = Y - \hat{\theta}_{OLS} X$ is the residual of the outcome after subtraction of the estimated observational association of the exposure. The sample size necessary for an IV analysis to demonstrate a given magnitude of causal effect is therefore approximately equal to that for a conventional epidemiological analysis to demonstrate the same magnitude of association divided by the parameter ρ_{GX}^2 for the IV [Wooldridge, 2009b]. As an example, if a genetic variant explains 2% of the variance in the exposure, then the sample size for a Mendelian randomization investigation is $1/0.02 = 50$ times that for a conventional epidemiological analysis.

This variance formula can be used to perform power calculations [Burgess, 2014]. We can calculate either: 1) the power to detect a particular magnitude of causal effect in a given sample size, or 2) the sample size needed to detect a particular magnitude of causal effect at a given power level. In both cases, the calculations require the proportion of variance in the exposure explained by the variants (ρ_{GX}^2), and the significance level. For a two-sample analysis, the relevant sample size is for the genetic associations with the outcome. With a binary outcome, the variance of the IV estimate also depends on the ratio of cases to controls. For a given sample size, power is maximized when the ratio is one case to one control. An online tool for performing power calculations is available at https://sb452.shinyapps.io/power/.

8.10   Choosing variants from a single gene region

Generally speaking, the choice of genetic variants to use in a Mendelian randomization analysis is a practical rather than a statistical issue. We discuss this issue at length in Section 10.3. Here, we suppose there is a single gene region of interest, and consider from a purely statistical perspective the question of selecting which variants to include from this gene region.

This scenario is particularly relevant for exposures that are molecular measurements, such as protein biomarkers or gene expression levels for a particular gene, for two reasons. First, these exposures often have a single relevant genetic region – the neighbourhood of the gene for gene expression, or the coding region for a protein. Such analyses been labelled as 'cis-Mendelian randomization analyses' [Schmidt et al., 2020], mirroring the terminology of cis (meaning 'close to') and trans (meaning 'far from') used in gene regulation to distinguish between variants near to the relevant gene from variants far from the relevant gene. Secondly, the proportion of variance explained by genetic variants is typically larger for exposures that are molecular measurements, meaning that it is often possible to find multiple variants in a single gene region that are independently associated with the exposure in a conditional model. In some cases, there are a large number (possibly hundreds) of genetic variants in and around the gene region of interest that are associated with the exposure and can be considered as candidate instruments.

If only a single variant is used in a Mendelian randomization analysis, then the analysis may be statistically inefficient. Variance explained (and hence power) can be increased by including multiple variants in the analysis that explain independent variation in the exposure, even if those variants are partially correlated (Section 5.2.6). But if too many genetic variants are included in the analysis, then collinearity between the variants can lead to numerical issues in estimation [Burgess et al., 2017c]. Therefore it is advised to perform pruning of variants to exclude highly correlated variants from the analysis [Yang et al., 2012]. A simple approach to do this is marginal stepwise pruning. First, select the genetic variant with the lowest p-value. Next, remove all other genetic variants from consideration that are correlated with the chosen variant at a given threshold correlation (say, $r^2 > 0.4$). Then, select the genetic variant with the lowest p-value from the remaining variants, and again remove variants correlated with the chosen variant. Repeat until all variants have been selected or removed, or no variants remain that are associated with the exposure at a given significance threshold. However, in some cases Mendelian randomization estimates have been shown to be sensitive to the choice of pruning thresholds [Burgess et al., 2017c].

Choosing which out of a set of highly correlated variants to include in a Mendelian randomization analysis is a topic of current methodological development. Two proposed solutions use principal components [Burgess et al., 2017c] or factor analysis [Patel et al., 2020] to perform dimension reduction on a set of variants, thus incorporating information on a large number of variants while avoiding both selection of variants and collinearity. Another approach uses Bayesian model averaging in a reversible jump Monte Carlo Markov chain implementation to average across estimates for different sets of variants [Gkatzionis et al., 2019].

8.11   Binary exposure

Use of a binary exposure complicates the interpretation of an IV estimate [Burgess and Labrecque, 2018]. Initially, we suppose that we have a valid IV for the binary exposure. This means that the only way that the IV can influence the outcome is via the binary exposure. If the IV changes, but the exposure stays the same, then the outcome should not change.

Monotonicity (Section 3.5.1) is the weaker of the assumptions needed for causal estimation, and means that we can define an exposure-increasing allele for each genetic variant such that for every individual in the population, having additional copies of the exposure-increasing allele increases their value of the exposure or keeps it constant. That is, there are no individuals in the population for whom having more copies of the exposure-increasing allele decreases their value of the exposure.

In a randomized controlled trial with a binary treatment, a 'complier' is an individual who complies with their allocation to treatment – they receive treatment if they are randomly assigned to take the treatment, and they do not receive treatment if they are randomly assigned to the control subgroup. The analogue of compliers in Mendelian randomization are individuals who would have the exposure present if they possess an exposure-increasing allele, but would not otherwise. Under the assumption of monotonicity, the IV estimate represents a complier-average causal effect, as it is the average effect of treatment (in a randomized controlled trial) or the exposure (in Mendelian randomization) in the compliers.

In well-designed randomized trials, compliers are likely to be common and may represent those who are likely to take the treatment in a real-world setting. Hence, compliers are a large and relevant subgroup of the population. However, as genetic variants typically do not explain a large proportion of variance in exposures, compliers in Mendelian randomization investigations are likely to be uncommon, and so the IV estimate represents the average causal estimate for a small and unrepresentative sample of the population. For example, suppose the exposure is vitamin D deficiency status, defined as present or absent based on a threshold cut-off. The IV estimate would be the average causal estimate in those individuals whose vitamin D deficiency status is influenced by the presence or absence of the genetic variants used in the Mendelian randomization analysis.

8.11.1   Binary exposure as dichotomization of a continuous risk factor

For most binary exposures used in Mendelian randomization investigations, there is an underlying continuous risk factor for which the binary variable is a dichotomization. For vitamin D deficiency, this is a dichotomization of the continuous risk factor vitamin D concentration. In more complex examples, an underlying continuous latent variable can be hypothesized even if it cannot be measured, such as a continuous spectrum of sub-clinical mental health problems for the binary exposure schizophrenia [Gage et al., 2017].

Such examples raise a practical issue of instrument validity for a binary exposure. Given that there is an arbitrary cutoff for defining a binary exposure such as vitamin D deficiency status, it is implausible that genetic predictors of vitamin D deficiency will be valid IVs for vitamin D deficiency status, as it is likely that increasing vitamin D levels (the continuous risk factor) could influence the outcome even if an individual's vitamin D deficiency status (the binary exposure) is unchanged. However, although the IV assumptions are technically violated in such a case, provided that the IV assumptions are satisfied for the underlying continuous risk factor, testing for an association with the outcome is still a valid test of the causal null hypothesis for the continuous risk factor.

There are two main consequences of this. First, a Mendelian randomization study for a dichotomous exposure should be conceptualized in terms of the underlying continuous risk factor, rather than the binary dichotomization of this variable. The IV assumptions should be assessed with the continuous risk factor in mind. Second, a causal estimate from a Mendelian randomization investigation with a dichotomized binary exposure does not have a clear interpretation due to the binary exposure variable not capturing the entirety of the causal relationship. An analysis using vitamin D deficiency status as the exposure should be interpreted as providing general evidence on vitamin D as a risk factor, and not on the specific dichotomized binary exposure of vitamin D deficiency.

8.11.2 Interpreting the causal estimate with a binary exposure

If the ratio or inverse-variance weighted method is performed using genetic associations (beta-coefficients) with a binary exposure estimated using logistic regression, then the literal interpretation of the IV estimate is the change in the outcome per unit increase in the log odds of the exposure. A unit increase in the log odds of a variable corresponds to a 2.72 (= exp 1)-fold multiplicative increase in the odds of the variable. If the exposure is rare, the odds of the exposure is approximately equal to the probability of the exposure. The causal estimate then represents the average change in the outcome per 2.72-fold increase in the prevalence of the exposure (for example, an increase in the exposure prevalence from 1% to 2.72%). It may be more interpretable to think instead about the average change in the outcome per doubling (2-fold increase) in the prevalence of the exposure. This can be obtained by multiplying the causal estimate by 0.693 (= $\log_e 2$).

8.11.3 Power with a binary exposure

If the genetic associations with the exposure are estimated using logistic regression, then conventional power calculations cannot be performed. This is because the power depends on the absolute change in the prevalence of the exposure, not the relative prevalence. As an example, increasing the exposure from a prevalence of 0.1% to 0.3% would represent the same change in the log odds of the exposure as an increase from 10% to 25%. However, the power to detect a causal effect will be much larger in the second case. A solution to this is to treat the binary exposure as a continuous variable and estimate genetic associations with the exposure using linear regression. Estimates could be expressed on an absolute scale for a fixed increase in the probability of the exposure (say, for a 10% absolute increase in the probability of the exposure). Power can be calculated for causal estimates expressed on this scale [Burgess and Labrecque, 2018].

8.12 Alternative estimation methods

While in this book we concentrate on the ratio, 2SLS, and inverse-variance weighted methods, there are other methods for performing IV analyses. We briefly mention the approach of calculating bounds for a causal effect, and describe the limited information maximum likelihood (LIML), and generalized method of moments (GMM), and structural mean model (SMM) methods. Other methods not discussed include the continuously updating estimation method [Davies et al., 2015], and Bayesian and other full-likelihood approaches [Burgess et al., 2010].

8.12.1   Bounds on the causal estimate

In Section 3.5.1, we stated that to estimate a causal effect, it was necessary to make assumptions of monotonicity or homogeneity. While this is true, without these additional conditions it is possible to calculate bounds for the average causal effect in the case of a binary exposure [Balke and Pearl, 1997]. In this case, these bounds can also be used to assess the validity of a genetic variant as an instrumental variable [Palmer et al., 2011b; Swanson et al., 2018]. However, these bounds are often so wide as to be uninformative in practice. Additionally, such bounds cannot be calculated for a continuous exposure.

8.12.2   Limited information maximum likelihood

LIML has been called the 'maximum likelihood counterpart of 2SLS' [Hayashi, 2000, page 227] and gives the same causal estimate as the 2SLS and ratio methods with a single IV. The LIML estimate can be intuitively understood as the value of the causal estimate that minimizes the residual sum of squares from the regression of the component of the outcome not caused by the exposure $(Y - \theta X)$ on the IVs. Informally, the LIML estimator is the causal parameter for which the component of the outcome not due to the exposure is as poorly predicted by the IVs as possible.

Use of LIML has been strongly discouraged by some, as LIML estimates do not have defined moments for any number of instruments [Hahn et al., 2004]. This means the bias of the method is not formally defined. However, its use has also been encouraged by others, especially with weak instruments, as the median of the distribution of the estimator is close to unbiased even with weak instruments [Angrist and Pischke, 2009a]. With large numbers of IVs (10 or more), standard confidence intervals from the LIML method with weak instruments are too narrow and a correction is needed (known as Bekker standard errors) [Bekker, 1994]. Although this correction is required to maintain nominal coverage levels, the efficiency of the LIML estimator is reduced, and it may be outperformed by a simple allele score approach [Davies et al., 2015].

8.12.3 Generalized method of moments and structural mean model methods

With the exception of the bounds discussed above, all methods previously considered in this book are parametric methods. They require full specification of the distribution of the variables in the analysis. In contrast, a semi-parametric method has both parametric and non-parametric components. Typically semi-parametric IV methods assume a parametric form for the equation relating the outcome and exposure (such as linearity or log-linearity), but make no assumption about the distribution of the errors. Semi-parametric models are designed to be more robust to model misspecification than fully parametric models [Clarke and Windmeijer, 2012].

The generalized method of moments (GMM) is a semi-parametric method designed as a more flexible form of 2SLS to deal with heteroscedasticity of error distributions and non-linearity in the second-stage structural model [Foster, 1997; Johnston et al., 2008]. With a single IV, the GMM estimate is chosen to give orthogonality between the IV and the residual values of the outcome after subtraction of the causal effect of the exposure. With multiple IVs, it is not possible for the correlation between the IV and the residuals to be simultaneously zero for all IVs, and so the GMM estimator minimizes an objective function based on all the orthogonality conditions [Hansen, 1982].

The structural mean model (SMM) approach is another semi-parametric estimation method developed in the context of randomized trials with incomplete compliance [Robins, 1994; Fischer-Lapp and Goetghebeur, 1999]. Here, the counterfactual values of the outcome are defined at different values of the exposure to be a parametric function of the exposure. Similarly to the GMM method, the estimator is chosen to give orthogonality between the IV and the counterfactual value of the outcome at a fixed value of the exposure (typically zero). For a continuous outcome, the GMM and SMM estimates are identical and coincide with the estimates from the ratio (for a single IV), 2SLS, and inverse-variance weighted methods [Palmer et al., 2011a]. For a binary outcome with a log-linear model, again the GMM and SMM estimates are identical. The methods only give different estimates for non-collapsible exposure–outcome models, such as a logistic model [Clarke and Windmeijer, 2012].

An advantage of the GMM and SMM methods is that they do not rely as strongly on parametric assumptions for effect estimation and for making inferences. A disadvantage is that the methods require access to individual-level data, and they are more difficult to implement in practice. In particular, there is no guarantee that the estimating equations for the methods have a unique solution [Burgess et al., 2014c]. This is especially likely if the IV is weak. We would therefore only recommend the methods to users who are confident in writing their own software code to perform and check optimization and convergence of estimating equations. While it is impossible to prove conclusively that issues such as departures from parametric linearity and normality assumptions are not serious reasons for bias and inflated Type 1 error rates, our experience from running numerous simulation studies is that parametric methods are generally robust to some deviation from the parametric assumptions, and issues such as instrument invalidity are likely to be a greater threat to inferences from IV analyses. For this reason, we consider other choices in performing a Mendelian randomization analysis more important than whether a fully parametric or semi-parametric method is used.

8.13   Summary

In summary, while we are not able to list all the factors that may influence a Mendelian randomization analysis, we have discussed the issues that are most likely to arise. Bias in a statistical analysis is not a binary phenomenon, and it would be a fallacy to think of biases such as weak instrument bias and collider bias as being either present or absent. Hence, pragmatic choices are necessary and judgement is required to design and perform the optimal analysis (or set of analyses) given the data available. In the next chapter, we discuss extensions to the standard Mendelian randomization paradigm, before returning in Chapter 10 to discuss practical aspects of making these choices in more detail.

9

Extensions to Mendelian randomization

In this chapter, we consider extensions to the basic Mendelian randomization paradigm. These include approaches with multiple exposure variables and those which aim to estimate a parameter other than that estimated in a standard Mendelian randomization investigation. We consider in turn multivariable Mendelian randomization, network Mendelian randomization, non-linear Mendelian randomization, factorial Mendelian randomization, bidirectional Mendelian randomization, and meta-analysis in Mendelian randomization.

9.1 Multivariable Mendelian randomization

Multivariable Mendelian randomization [Burgess and Thompson, 2015] is an extension to standard Mendelian randomization that can be used when it is difficult to find genetic variants specifically and uniquely associated with a particular exposure, but it is possible to find genetic variants specifically associated with a set of related exposures. For example, it is difficult to find genetic variants associated with HDL-cholesterol that are not also associated with LDL-cholesterol and triglycerides [Burgess et al., 2014b]. In multivariable Mendelian randomization, genetic variants are allowed to be associated with more than one exposure, as long as they are not associated with confounders of any of the exposure–outcome associations and they do not directly affect the outcome – that is, any genetic association with the outcome is mediated via one or more of the exposures.

The instrumental variable (IV) assumptions for a genetic variant in multivariable Mendelian randomization are:

i. the variant is associated with one or more of the exposures,

ii. the variant is not associated with the outcome via a confounding pathway, and

iii. the variant does not affect the outcome directly, only possibly indirectly via one or more of the exposures.

These assumptions are similar to those for standard Mendelian randomization (Section 3.2.1), except that they are expressed with respect to multiple exposures. A directed acyclic graph illustrating the assumptions is presented in Figure 9.1. Although the diagram has arrows from all the genetic variants to each of the exposures, it is not necessary for each variant to be associated with every exposure. However, each exposure must be associated with at least one genetic variant.

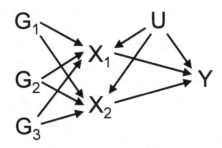

FIGURE 9.1

Directed acyclic graph of multivariable Mendelian randomization assumptions for three genetic variants G_1, G_2, G_3, two exposures X_1, X_2, and outcome Y. Confounders U are assumed to be unknown.

Standard (that is, univariable) Mendelian randomization assesses whether genetically-predicted values of the exposure are associated with the outcome. Multivariable Mendelian randomization assesses whether genetically-predicted values of multiple exposures are associated with the outcome in a multivariable model. The technique relies on some genetic variants being more strongly associated with some exposures than with others [Sanderson et al., 2019]. For example, although most genetic predictors of body mass index influence both fat mass and fat-free mass, some variants influence fat mass proportionally more strongly, and others influence fat-free mass more strongly. Hence, multivariable Mendelian randomization can be used to disentangle the causal effects of fat mass and fat-free mass [Larsson et al., 2020]. Formally, to ensure the causal effects of each exposure can be identified, some degree of linear independence is needed in the genetically-predicted values of the exposures (for individual-level data) or equivalently in the genetic associations with the exposures (for summarized data). If the genetic associations with two exposures are collinear, then it is not possible to distinguish which is the causal risk factor. This means that the number of genetic variants in a multivariable Mendelian randomization analysis must be at least as many as the number of exposures.

9.1.1 Implementing multivariable Mendelian randomization

With individual-level data, multivariable Mendelian randomization can be implemented using the two-stage least squares method (for a continuous outcome) or the relevant two-stage method (for other outcomes) (Section 4.2). We illustrate the method for a continuous outcome.

In the first stage, we regress each exposure variable on all the genetic variants. In the second stage, we regress the outcome on fitted values of the exposure variables in a multivariable regression model. Indexing individuals by i, genetic variants by j, and exposures by k, the regression models are:

$$x_{ik} = \beta_{0k} + \sum_j \beta_{jk} g_{ij} + \varepsilon_{Xik} \quad \text{for } k = 1, \ldots, K \tag{9.1}$$

$$y_i = \theta_0 + \sum_k \theta_k \hat{x}_{ik} + \varepsilon_{Yi} \tag{9.2}$$

where $\hat{x}_{ik}$ are the fitted values of the kth exposure from the corresponding first-stage regression, and θ_k is the multivariable Mendelian randomization causal effect parameter for the kth exposure.

With summarized data on the univariate associations of genetic variants with each exposure in turn ($\hat{\beta}_{Xj1}, \hat{\beta}_{Xj2}, \ldots, \hat{\beta}_{XjK}$ for each variant $j = 1, 2, \ldots, J$ with each exposure $k = 1, 2, \ldots, K$), and genetic associations with the outcome (estimate $\hat{\beta}_{Yj}$, standard error $\text{se}(\hat{\beta}_{Yj})$) for each variant j, the inverse-variance weighted method can be extended to a multivariable weighted regression model:

$$\hat{\beta}_{Yj} = \theta_1 \hat{\beta}_{Xj1} + \theta_2 \hat{\beta}_{Xj2} + \cdots + \theta_K \hat{\beta}_{XjK} + \varepsilon_j, \quad \varepsilon_j \sim \mathcal{N}(0, \text{se}(\hat{\beta}_{Yj})^2) \tag{9.3}$$

As for univariable Mendelian randomization, it can be shown that the multivariable two-stage least squares (2SLS) and inverse-variance weighted (IVW) estimates are identical with a continuous outcome and uncorrelated genetic variants [Burgess et al., 2015b]. The multivariable IVW method can be extended to allow for correlated variants using generalized weighted regression in a similar way to the univariable case [Burgess et al., 2017b] (Section 5.2.6). There is also a corresponding multivariable MR-Egger method that accounts for unmeasured pleiotropy by including an intercept term in equation (9.3) [Rees et al., 2017], as well as a multivariable median-based method and a multivariable version of the MR-Lasso method [Grant and Burgess, 2020b].

The relevant measure of instrument strength in a multivariable Mendelian randomization analysis is the expected conditional F statistic, representing the strength of association of the genetic variants with each exposure conditional on all other exposures in the analysis [Sanderson and Windmeijer, 2016].

The 2SLS method can be implemented for multivariable Mendelian randomization using the same computer packages as for univariable Mendelian randomization (Section 4.4). The multivariable IVW method can be implemented in R using the `mr_mvivw` command in the *MendelianRandomization* package available from the Comprehensive R Archive Network (CRAN) [Yavorska and Burgess, 2017]. The syntax is:

```
mr_mvivw(mr_mvinput(bx, bxse, by, byse))
```

where `bx` and `bxse` are matrices of the genetic associations with the exposures.

9.1.2   Multivariable Mendelian randomization and mediation

It can be shown that the parameters $\theta_1, \theta_2, \ldots, \theta_K$ estimated in multivariable Mendelian randomization represent the direct causal effects of each exposure in turn on the outcome [Sanderson et al., 2019]. The direct effect of an exposure represents the change in the outcome when intervening on the exposure of interest while keeping all other exposures fixed. As a technical aside, while there are several versions of direct effects depending on the value that other exposures are fixed to take, when the effects of the exposures are linear and homogeneous in the population, these are numerically identical [Burgess et al., 2017b].

This provides a second motivation for the use of multivariable Mendelian randomization. The estimate from standard (that is, univariable) Mendelian randomization represents the total effect of the exposure on the outcome. When both analyses are based on the same variants, if estimates differ for univariable Mendelian randomization of an exposure on the outcome, and multivariable Mendelian randomization for the exposure and another trait, then there are two explanations: the trait is on a pleiotropic pathway from the genetic variants to the outcome, or the trait is a mediator on the causal pathway from the genetic variants to the outcome via the exposure (Figure 9.2) [Grant and Burgess, 2020a]. In the second case, if the genetic associations with the mediator are entirely mediated via the exposure in a homogeneous and linear way, then they will become perfectly correlated with the genetic associations with the exposure as the sample size increases, and multivariable Mendelian randomization will not be possible. However, if either some variants have pleiotropic effects on the mediator, or else there is heterogeneity between individuals in the effect of the exposure on the mediator, then multivariable Mendelian randomization will provide a meaningful estimate of the direct effect of the exposure [Burgess et al., 2017b].

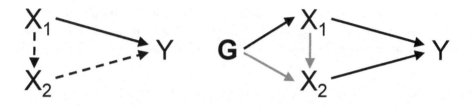

FIGURE 9.2

Directed acyclic graphs illustrating direct and indirect effects for two exposures X_1 and X_2 and an outcome Y. In the left diagram, the total effect of X_1 on Y comprises a direct effect (solid arrow) and an indirect effect via X_2 (dashed arrows). In the right diagram, if genetic variants **G** only affect X_1, then the total effect of X_1 can be estimated using standard (univariable) Mendelian randomization. Bold face is used for **G** to indicate that multiple genetic variants are required to perform the multivariable analysis. If the multivariable estimate differs from the univariable estimate, then either there is a pleiotropic pathway from at least one element of **G** to X_2 or there is a causal effect of X_1 on X_2 (grey arrows). In either case, the multivariable estimate represents the direct effect of X_1 on Y (that is, the effect not via X_2).

As an example, when considering the causal effect of age at menarche on breast cancer risk, univariable Mendelian randomization suggested a null total effect of age at menarche on breast cancer risk (odds ratio per 1 year later menarche 1.00, 95% confidence interval 0.96 to 1.05) [Burgess et al., 2017b]. However, a multivariable Mendelian randomization analysis adjusting for genetic associations with body mass index (BMI) indicated a protective direct effect of later age at menarche (odds ratio 0.94, 95% confidence interval 0.89 to 0.98). This suggests that an intervention to delay menarche would have no net effect on breast cancer risk if it also had the expected consequence of lowering BMI: this represents the total effect of menarche on breast cancer risk. However, an intervention which had an effect on post-pubertal sex-hormone exposure equivalent to a later menarche would be likely to have a protective effect on breast cancer risk. As such an intervention could not affect pubertal timing and hence would not alter BMI, only the direct effect of age at menarche on breast cancer risk (that is, the effect of exposure to sex-hormones) would apply.

Multivariable Mendelian randomization is an active area of research, driven by the increasing availability of high-dimensional sets of variables. Recent extensions include methods for variable selection amongst large numbers of exposure variables [Zuber et al., 2020], consideration of multiple mediators in a single model [Carter et al., 2019b], and multiple measures of the same exposure at different timepoints [Richardson et al., 2020].

9.2 Network Mendelian randomization

An alternative approach for assessing mediation in a Mendelian randomization setting is network Mendelian randomization [Burgess et al., 2015a]. Assuming linearity and homogeneity of effects, the total effect of the exposure on the outcome should equal the direct effect of the exposure on the outcome plus the indirect effect via the mediator. This indirect effect can be expressed as the effect of the exposure on the mediator multiplied by the effect of the mediator on the outcome:

$$\theta_{X \to Y} = \theta_{X \Rightarrow Y} + \theta_{X \to Z}\, \theta_{Z \to Y}, \tag{9.4}$$

where X is the exposure, Z is the mediator, Y is the outcome, $\to$ represents a total causal effect and $\Rightarrow$ represents a direct effect [Carter et al., 2019b]. If separate IVs are available for the exposure and a mediator (Figure 9.3), then the direct effect of the exposure on the outcome can be estimated by a difference method:

$$\hat{\theta}_{X \Rightarrow Y} = \hat{\theta}_{X \to Y} - \hat{\theta}_{X \to Z}\, \hat{\theta}_{Z \to Y}, \tag{9.5}$$

as all the quantities on the right-hand side of the equation are total effects and so can be estimated by separate IV analyses. While it is also possible to use this formula to calculate an indirect effect, the formal definition of an indirect effect is somewhat complex, and so we recommend that Mendelian randomization investigations should concentrate on comparisons between direct and total effects.

A multivariable approach to investigating mediation was used in the case of age at menarche and breast cancer (Section 9.1.2), as for this analysis we were not primarily interested in the effect of BMI, but only insofar as it mediates the effect of age at menarche. Other mechanisms by which BMI may influence breast cancer risk are not relevant to the investigation. Hence, we only included in the multivariable analysis genetic variants that are associated with age at menarche. To implement multivariable Mendelian randomization with summarized data, we required the genetic associations of all variants with both age at menarche and breast cancer risk. In contrast, the network approach requires separate IVs for the exposure and the mediator, and estimates effects of the exposure and mediator in separate analyses.

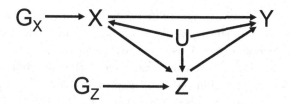

FIGURE 9.3

Directed acyclic graph illustrating network Mendelian randomization. Genetic variants G_X can be used to estimate the total causal effect of the exposure X on the outcome Y, as well as the causal effect of X on the mediator Z. Genetic variants G_Z can be used to estimate the causal effect of the mediator Z on the outcome Y. The direct effect of X on Y that does not pass through Z can be calculated by the difference method.

9.3 Non-linear Mendelian randomization

In some cases, the causal effect of the exposure on the outcome may be non-linear. It may be that the causal relationship between the exposure and outcome has a threshold shape, meaning that increases in the exposure only affect the outcome above or below a threshold value. Or that increases in the exposure have a larger average impact on the outcome for individuals with higher or lower values of the exposure. In some cases, the causal effect of the exposure on the outcome may be non-monotone (that is, increases in the exposure may increase the outcome on average for one subgroup of the population, but decrease it for another subgroup). Examples of non-monotone causal relationships are J-shaped and U-shaped relationships. We ask two questions: first, if the true causal relationship between the exposure and outcome is non-linear, how to interpret a causal estimate that makes an assumption of linearity? And second, how can the shape of the causal relationship be estimated?

If several genetic variants are available that have large effects on the exposure, then the shape of the causal relationship between the exposure and outcome can be assessed directly. Returning to the example of lipoprotein(a) and coronary heart disease risk (Section 6.3), Figure 6.2 showed that genetic associations with lipoprotein(a) and log odds of coronary heart disease risk were approximately proportional for several variants. This suggests that a log-linear relationship is a reasonable model across the observed range of genetic associations with lipoprotein(a), which was up to 70 mg/dL (for reference, the median lipoprotein(a) concentration in the population was around 30 mg/dL). However, for most exposures considered in Mendelian randomization, such a large range of genetic associations is not available.

As genetic variants are typically associated with small differences relative to the range of the distribution of an exposure, Mendelian randomization estimates usually reflect the predicted impact of a shift in the distribution of the exposure averaged across the population. As an example, the rs1421085 variant (located in the *FTO* gene region) was shown in a previous genome-wide association study to explain the most variation in BMI of any single variant [Speliotes et al., 2010]. The variant has an association with BMI of 0.6 kg/m^2 per additional allele, whereas BMI typically ranges from about 17 to 40 kg/m^2. A density plot of the distribution of BMI in genetically-defined subgroups of the population according to this variant is shown in Figure 9.4. So a Mendelian randomization analysis using this genetic variant would compare subgroups which differ only slightly in their average level of BMI. Non-linearities on this reduced scale would not be apparent, and thus standard (that is, linear) Mendelian randomization would not address many clinically relevant questions, such as about the potential harm of reducing BMI in underweight individuals.

The estimate from a linear IV analysis, such as the ratio method, represents a population-averaged causal effect [Angrist et al., 1996]. If the exposure–outcome relationship is not monotone, then the true change in the outcome for a given change in the exposure may be in different directions for different individuals in the population. In such a case, the IV estimate, representing the average change in the outcome across the population, would average over negative and positive effects [Angrist et al., 2000]. However, it will only be equal to zero if the causal effect is zero for all individuals in the population, or in the extremely unlikely case that negative and positive effects on average exactly balance out. Hence, standard IV methods can still be used to test for the presence of a causal effect even if the exposure–outcome relationship is non-linear. The IV estimate does have an interpretation, and potentially a relevant interpretation if investigators are interested in shifting the distribution of the exposure, but any single effect estimate will not necessarily tell the whole story.

While extrapolation of a Mendelian randomization estimate to a larger change in the exposure than is associated with the genetic variants should generally be avoided, it is particularly unwise when the exposure–outcome relationship is not monotone, as the genetic variants are not informative about the impact of a larger shift in the distribution of the exposure in the population (Section 6.1.3).

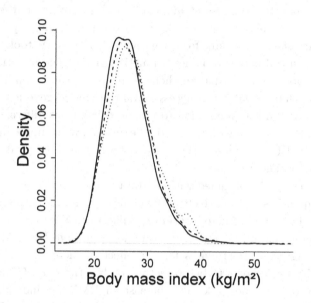

FIGURE 9.4

Distribution of body mass index in subgroups of the EPIC-InterAct study defined by genetic variant rs1421085: solid line – major homozygotes; dashed line – heterozygotes; dotted line – minor homozygotes. Densities are smoothed using a kernel-density method with a common bandwidth. Taken from Burgess et al. [2014a].

9.3.1   Localized average causal effects

In a classical epidemiological analysis, the shape of the association between the exposure and outcome can be approximated by stratifying on the exposure. In Mendelian randomization, direct stratification on the exposure is not possible, as the exposure is a mediator on the causal pathway from the genetic variants to the outcome, and a collider between the genetic variants and the confounders (Section 8.5). Instead, we initially subtract the effect of the IV on the exposure from the exposure measurement to obtain the 'IV-free exposure' or 'residual exposure' [Burgess et al., 2014a]. This quantity is the residual from regression of the exposure on the genetic variants, and represents the expected value of the exposure for an individual if their IV took the value zero. As the residual exposure is not a function of the genetic variants, it is neither a mediator nor a collider, and hence can then be safely conditioned on. For this approach to be valid, it is necessary for the average genetic association with the exposure in the population to remain constant at different levels of the exposure. By stratifying on the residual exposure, we compare individuals who, if they had the same genotype, would be in the same stratum of the exposure distribution (Figure 9.5).

IV estimates can be obtained within strata of the residual exposure, such as deciles or quintiles. Alternatively, more clinically relevant cutpoints for the exposure can be chosen. These stratum-specific estimates are referred to as 'localized average causal effects'. For example, in a large UK-based cohort, localized average causal estimates for the effect of increasing BMI on all-cause mortality were shown to be protective (odds ratio 0.57, 95% confidence interval, 0.41 to 0.79, per 1 kg/m^2 increase in BMI) for individuals with residual BMI in the underweight category (residual BMI < 18.5 kg/m^2), but harmful (odds ratio 1.11, 95% confidence interval 1.05 to 1.18) for individuals with residual BMI in the obese category (residual BMI $\geq$ 30.0 kg/m^2) [Sun et al., 2019b]. The plot in Figure 9.6 (top panel) shows the associations of an allele score for BMI with all-cause mortality in 30 strata of the population defined according to residual BMI. Estimates in the lowest strata are negative, whereas estimates in strata with mean BMI above 23 are generally positive. This suggests that the causal relationship between BMI and all-cause mortality is J-shaped. However, the protective effect of increasing BMI in the underweight category was not evident when restricting the analysis to never-smokers, suggesting that this protective effect in underweight individuals may be limited to ever-smokers.

In estimating localized average causal effects, there is a trade-off between a fine stratification into a large number of quantile groups, and a coarse stratification into a small number of groups [Burgess et al., 2014a]. A large

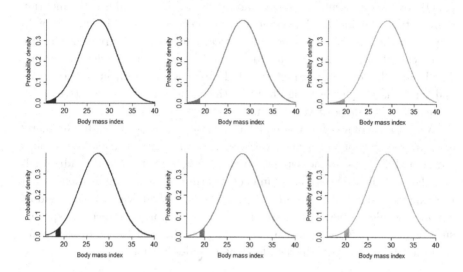

FIGURE 9.5

Synthetic data for the population distribution of an exposure (here, body mass index, kg/m²) to illustrate estimation of localized average causal effects in two strata of the population for a single genetic variant which is a biallelic SNP. The left column represents individuals with zero copies of the variant allele, the middle column represents one copy, and the right column represents two copies. By stratifying on the residual exposure, we calculate an IV estimate that compares the shaded groups. The top row corresponds to the lowest stratum of the residual exposure. The bottom row corresponds to the next lowest stratum. Continuing in this way, separate IV estimates (referred to as 'localized average causal effects') can be obtained for each stratum of the population defined by the residual exposure.

number of groups enables a more detailed estimate of the shape of the relationship, but the estimates in each stratum will be less precise. A fractional polynomial method has been developed which allows smoothing over large numbers of strata to estimate the causal relationship in a flexible parametric framework [Staley and Burgess, 2017]. A figure showing the output from this method for BMI and all-cause mortality is displayed in Figure 9.6 (bottom panel). To be consistent with a standard epidemiological analysis, the function representing the localized average causal effect has been integrated with respect to the exposure, so that the vertical axis does not represent the size of the causal effect, but the hazard ratio with respect to a reference group. The localized average causal effect is indicated by the gradient of the graph, and the J-shaped plot here signifies that the causal estimate is negative at low values of BMI, but positive at higher values.

A limitation of non-linear Mendelian randomization is that individual-level data are required on the genetic variants, exposure, and outcome in the same individuals (a one-sample setting). This is necessary to stratify individuals and then calculate IV estimates in each stratum. A further limitation is that the exposure must be truly continuous, otherwise stratifying on the residual exposure would be the same as stratifying on the exposure. Hence an exposure such as age at menarche, which is typically only known to the nearest year, could not be used in non-linear Mendelian randomization.

9.4   Factorial Mendelian randomization

Factorial Mendelian randomization is the use of genetic variants to answer questions about interactions [Rees et al., 2019a]. It is named in analogy to a factorial randomized trial. The approach has been considered in two broad scenarios: 1) to estimate causal effect interactions between exposures by using genetic variants as predictors of the exposures; and 2) to identify interactions between interventions by using genetic variants as proxies for specific treatments. In the first case, the aim is to identify an interaction between the causal effects of two (or more) distinct exposures on the outcome. In the second case, the aim is to identify an interaction between the interventions for which the genetic variants are proxies.

The first scenario can be seen as an extension of multivariable Mendelian randomization. If there are two exposures, we can additionally estimate an interaction term in the second-stage of the 2SLS method:

$$y_i = \theta_0 + \theta_1 \hat{x}_{i1} + \theta_2 \hat{x}_{i2} + \theta_{12} \hat{x}_{i12} + \varepsilon_i \qquad (9.6)$$

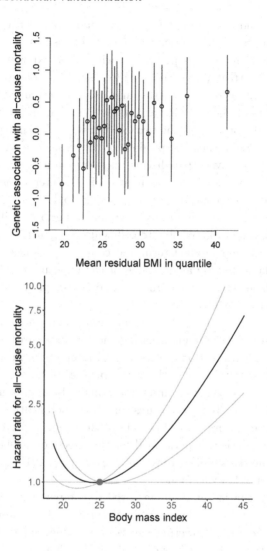

FIGURE 9.6

Non-linear causal relationship between BMI (kg/m^2) and all-cause mortality in a UK-based cohort. Top panel: Genetic associations with all-cause mortality (log hazard ratio per unit increase in allele score) estimated within strata of the population defined according to residual BMI. Error bars represent 95% confidence intervals. Bottom panel: Causal relationship estimated using fractional polynomial method. The gradient at each point of the curve is the localized average causal effect. Hazard ratios are expressed relative to a BMI of 25 kg/m^2. Grey lines represent 95% confidence intervals. Taken from Sun et al. [2019b].

where i indexes individuals and θ_{12} is the interaction term, the coefficient for the fitted values of the product of the two exposures $x_{i12} = x_{i1}x_{i2}$. The multivariable 2SLS method is performed with three exposures: the product of the exposures is treated as a separate exposure variable. In the first-stage regression, in addition to the genetic variants, it is recommended to use the pairwise products of the genetic variants as IVs. This is to better estimate fitted values for the product of the two exposures, as if each exposure is linear in the genetic variants, then the product of the exposures will be a function of these cross-terms. Even though this may lead to a large number of IVs, simulations have suggested that estimates of the interaction term are not sensitive to weak instrument bias [Rees et al., 2019a].

Factorial Mendelian randomization cannot be performed if only standard summarized data are available, due to collinearity of genetic associations with the exposures and their product term, but could be performed if summarized data were available for the associations of the exposures and their product term with each genetic variant and each pairwise product of the genetic variants [Rees et al., 2019a].

If the interaction term differs from zero, then there is a statistical interaction present in the model relating the two exposures to the outcome. This could indicate a functional or biological interaction, in which there is a mechanistic connection between the two exposures in how they influence the outcome. However, a statistical interaction may also represent non-linearity in the effect of one or both exposures, or effect modification, meaning that the effect of one exposure varies in strata of the other. A factorial Mendelian randomization analysis was performed for the effects of alcohol consumption and obesity on markers of liver function [Carter et al., 2019a]; no evidence for a statistical interaction was found.

The second scenario has been employed to compare the effect of lowering LDL-cholesterol levels on the log odds of coronary heart disease using two different LDL-cholesterol lowering agents (ezetimibe and statin), compared with a combination of both [Ference et al., 2015]. Genetic variants associated with LDL-cholesterol were identified in the *NPC1L1* gene (proxies for ezetimibe), and the *HMGCR* gene (proxies for statins), and combined into separate allele scores. To mimic a 2×2 factorial randomized trial, the two allele scores were dichotomized to create a 2×2 contingency table (Figure 9.7). The allele scores were dichotomized at their median values so that the numbers of participants were balanced across the four groups. The 2×2 contingency table can also be used to illustrate a factorial Mendelian randomization investigation for distinct exposures. In this example, no interaction was found, providing no evidence against the hypothesis that the effects of ezetimibe and statin on coronary heart disease risk are linear and additive on the log odds scale.

Factorial randomized trial		Randomization of A	
		Control	Treatment A
Randomization of B	Control	Incidence under usual care	Incidence under intervention in A
	Treatment B	Incidence under intervention in B	Incidence under intervention in A and B

Factorial Mendelian randomization for two exposures		Genetic score 1	
		Below median	Above median
Genetic score 2	Below median	Incidence with exposure 1 lower, exposure 2 lower	Incidence with exposure 1 higher, exposure 2 lower
	Above median	Incidence with exposure 1 lower, exposure 2 higher	Incidence with exposure 1 higher, exposure 2 higher

Factorial Mendelian randomization for two interventions		Genetic score 1	
		Below median	Above median
Genetic score 2	Below median	Incidence with no proxied treatment	Incidence under genetically-proxied treatment A
	Above median	Incidence under genetically-proxied treatment B	Incidence under genetically-proxied treatments A and B

FIGURE 9.7

Comparison of a factorial randomized trial and a factorial Mendelian randomization investigation with a 2 × 2 approach. Top panel: factorial randomized trial for two treatments; middle panel: factorial Mendelian randomization for two exposures; bottom panel: factorial Mendelian randomization for two interventions on the same exposure.

While framing the analysis in a 2×2 table is convenient way of presenting results, dichotomizing variables can reduce power [Rees et al., 2019a]. Instead, investigators could have calculated a weighted allele score for each set of variants based on their associations with the target of intervention (in this case, LDL-cholesterol), and regressed the outcome on these two scores and their product. Again, a statistical interaction would be evidenced if the coefficient for the product term differed from zero.

9.5   Bidirectional Mendelian randomization

In some situations, the direction of the causal effect between the exposure and outcome may be unclear. Bidirectional Mendelian randomization assesses the effect of the exposure on the outcome, but also the effect of the outcome on the exposure [Burgess et al., 2015a]. For this to be possible, it is necessary to have genetic variants that are IVs for the exposure and separately genetic variants that are IVs for the outcome (Figure 9.8). This may be difficult to achieve in practice, as if there truly are bidirectional causal effects between the exposure and the outcome, then any genetic predictor of the exposure will also be associated with the outcome and vice versa. It is necessary to identify which genetic variants influence the exposure primarily, and which influence the outcome primarily.

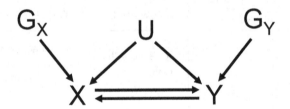

FIGURE 9.8
Directed graph illustrating bidirectional Mendelian randomization. Genetic variants G_X can be used to estimate the causal effect of the exposure X on the outcome Y. Genetic variants G_Y can be used to estimate the causal effect of the outcome Y on the exposure X.

An example of bidirectional Mendelian randomization concerns the causal relationship between education and myopia [Mountjoy et al., 2018]. It has long been noted that individuals who spend a long time studying are more likely to have problems with their eyesight. However, it was not clear whether excess study causes shortsightedness, or whether becoming shortsighted makes an individual more likely to spend time studying (reverse causation). Bidirectional Mendelian randomization indicated clear evidence for directionality: genetic predictors of spending longer in education were associated with increases in shortsightedness, whereas genetic predictors of shortsightedness were not associated with spending longer in education.

It is possible for bidirectional Mendelian randomization investigations to suggest causal effects in both directions. In this case, contextual judgement is required to understand how the traits are related. For example, genetic predictors of BMI associate with increased smoking prevalence (perhaps smokers seeking to reduce weight) [Carreras-Torres et al., 2018], but genetic predictors of cigarette smoking associate with decreased BMI (as cigarette smoking is an appetite suppressant) [Taylor et al., 2018]. This suggests that high BMI causes people to smoke more, but smoking more causes reductions in BMI.

Interpretation of causal effects in a bidirectional Mendelian randomization analysis requires a high degree of confidence in the genetic variants used as IVs for the exposure and the outcome. Investigators will have to convincingly argue that the genetic associations with the causal descendent (the claimed downstream affected variable) only occur due to the effect of the causal antecedent (the claimed upstream causal factor).

9.6 Mendelian randomization and meta-analysis

A final situation which goes beyond a standard Mendelian randomization analysis is when data are combined from multiple sources. Estimates from multiple studies can be combined using standard methods from the meta-analysis literature, such as inverse-variance weighting. When data are available on multiple genetic variants from multiple studies, investigators have a choice whether to combine data on the genetic associations within the studies into study-specific causal estimates, which can then be combined by meta-analysis, or to combine data on the genetic associations for each variant across studies into variant-specific genetic associations, which can then be combined using the IVW method. Combining genetic associations across studies for each variant is recommended if investigators are particularly interested in investigating heterogeneity between the variant-specific causal estimates.

Calculating causal estimates across variants within studies is recommended if investigators are more concerned about between-study heterogeneity.

9.7   Summary

In summary, Mendelian randomization provides a framework for using genetic variants as proxy measurements for an exposure to assess the impact on an outcome of an intervention in the exposure. This chapter has demonstrated how this framework can be exploited in various ways beyond simply considering the causal effect of a single exposure variable. In the next chapter, we bring together the various methods and issues that have been introduced in this and previous chapters, and provide practical advice on how to perform a Mendelian randomization investigation.

10

How to perform a Mendelian randomization investigation

In previous chapters, we have described methods for estimating causal effects using Mendelian randomization, and discussed issues that can arise when performing a Mendelian randomization analysis. The aim of this chapter is to provide practical guidelines for performing Mendelian randomization investigations.

These guidelines are deliberately written as suggestions and recommendations rather than as prescriptive rules, as we believe that there is no recipe or single 'right way' to perform a Mendelian randomization investigation. Best practice will depend on the aim of the investigation and the specific exposure and outcome variables. While it is not possible to cover every possible eventuality, we hope these guidelines will help investigators to consider the key issues in designing, undertaking, presenting, and reviewing Mendelian randomization analyses. The guidelines in this chapter are summarized from a position paper written by several leading researchers in the field [Burgess et al., 2020a].

A flowchart highlighting some of the key analytic steps and choices is provided in Figure 10.1, and a one-page checklist summarizing these guidelines is provided in Figure 10.2. The guidelines are divided into nine sections: motivation and scope, data sources, choice of genetic variants, variant harmonization, primary analysis, supplementary and sensitivity analyses (one section on robust methods and one on other approaches), data presentation, and interpretation.

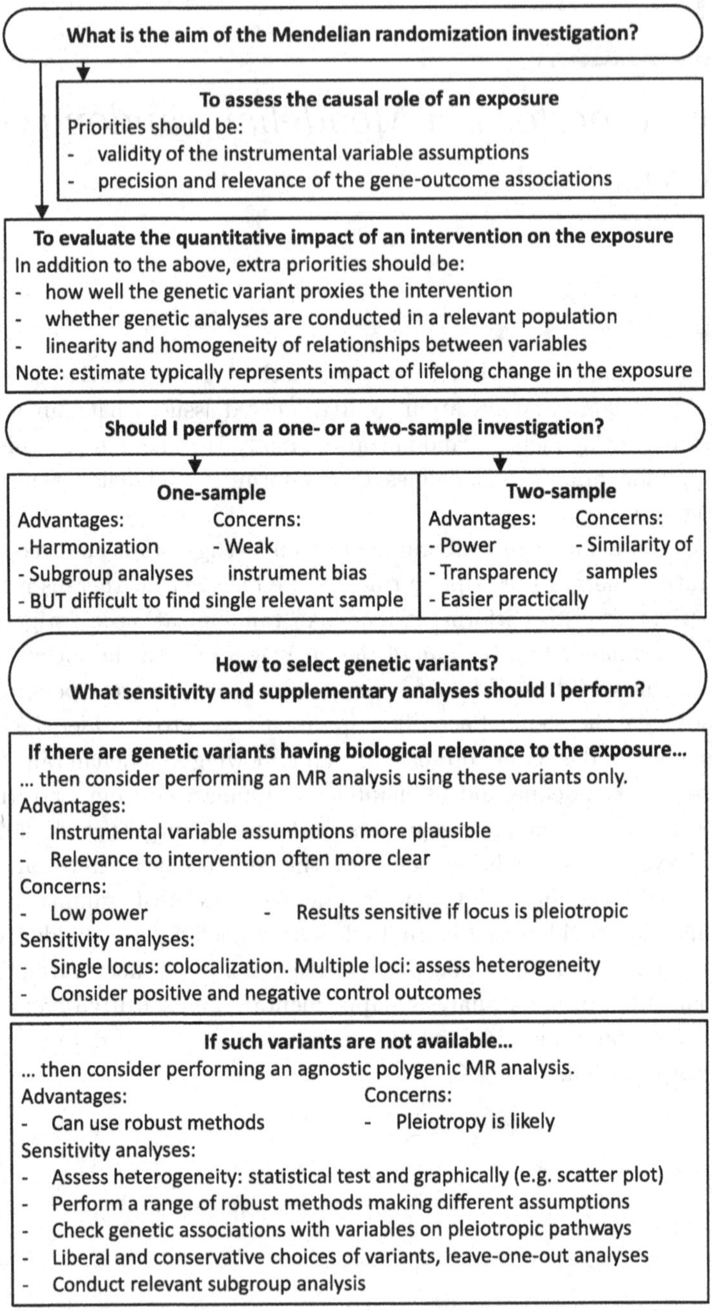

What is the aim of the Mendelian randomization investigation?

To assess the causal role of an exposure
Priorities should be:
- validity of the instrumental variable assumptions
- precision and relevance of the gene-outcome associations

To evaluate the quantitative impact of an intervention on the exposure
In addition to the above, extra priorities should be:
- how well the genetic variant proxies the intervention
- whether genetic analyses are conducted in a relevant population
- linearity and homogeneity of relationships between variables
Note: estimate typically represents impact of lifelong change in the exposure

Should I perform a one- or a two-sample investigation?

One-sample		**Two-sample**	
Advantages:	Concerns:	Advantages:	Concerns:
- Harmonization	- Weak	- Power	- Similarity of
- Subgroup analyses	instrument bias	- Transparency	samples
- BUT difficult to find single relevant sample		- Easier practically	

How to select genetic variants?
What sensitivity and supplementary analyses should I perform?

If there are genetic variants having biological relevance to the exposure...
... then consider performing an MR analysis using these variants only.
Advantages:
- Instrumental variable assumptions more plausible
- Relevance to intervention often more clear
Concerns:
- Low power   - Results sensitive if locus is pleiotropic
Sensitivity analyses:
- Single locus: colocalization. Multiple loci: assess heterogeneity
- Consider positive and negative control outcomes

If such variants are not available...
... then consider performing an agnostic polygenic MR analysis.
Advantages: Concerns:
- Can use robust methods   - Pleiotropy is likely
Sensitivity analyses:
- Assess heterogeneity: statistical test and graphically (e.g. scatter plot)
- Perform a range of robust methods making different assumptions
- Check genetic associations with variables on pleiotropic pathways
- Liberal and conservative choices of variants, leave-one-out analyses
- Conduct relevant subgroup analysis

FIGURE 10.1
Flowchart highlighting some of the key analytic choices in performing a Mendelian randomization (MR) analysis.

Checklist for reviewing Mendelian randomization investigations

1. What is the primary hypothesis of interest? What is the motivation for using Mendelian randomization? What is the scope of the investigation? What and how many primary analyses?

2. Data sources

    What type of Mendelian randomization investigation is this? One-sample or two-sample? Sample overlap? Summarized data or individual-level data? Drawn from same population? Relevance to applied research?

3. Selection of genetic variants – how were the genetic variants chosen? Single or multiple gene regions?
    a. Biological rationale?
    b. GWAS analysis? If so, what dataset? What was the *p*-value threshold? Clumping?
    c. Were genetic variants excluded from the analysis? Associations with pleiotropic pathways?
    d. How else was the validity of genetic variants as instrumental variables assessed?

4. Variant harmonization (for two-sample analyses)

    Was it checked that genetic variants were appropriately orientated across the datasets?

5. Primary analysis

    What was the primary analysis? What was the statistical method? How implemented? Multiple testing?

6 and 7.   Supplementary and sensitivity analyses

    What analyses were performed to support and assess the validity of the primary analysis?
    For example: stricter criteria for variant selection, assess heterogeneity, robust methods, subgroup analysis, positive/negative controls, 'leave-one-out' analyses, colocalization (single gene region)

8. Data presentation

    How are the data and results presented to allow readers to assess the analysis and assumptions?
    For example: scatter plot, forest/funnel/radial plot, R^2/F statistics, comparison of methods, power

9. Interpretation

    How have results been interpreted, particularly any numerical estimates?

FIGURE 10.2

Checklist of questions to consider when reading a Mendelian randomization investigation. A printable version of these guidelines can be found at http://www.mendelianrandomization.com/images/guidelines.pdf.

10.1   Motivation and scope

Mendelian randomization uses genetic variants to assess evidence for causal relationships in observational data. Before embarking on a Mendelian randomization analysis, investigators should consider the aims of their investigation and the primary hypothesis of interest. There are many potential motivations for using Mendelian randomization, and the motivation should influence decisions on how to perform the analysis, and how to arrange and present its results. The objective of a Mendelian randomization analysis is typically to test a causal hypothesis, and often additionally to estimate a causal effect (Sections 3.3 and 3.5).

If a Mendelian randomization investigation is performed primarily to assess whether an exposure has a causal effect on an outcome, then estimating the size of the causal effect of the exposure on the outcome is less important and may even be unnecessary [Didelez and Sheehan, 2007; VanderWeele et al., 2014]. For example, Mendelian randomization has demonstrated a causal effect of time spent in education during childhood on Alzheimer's disease [Larsson et al., 2017b]. However, those at risk of Alzheimer's disease are unable to extend their time in education. The analysis tests a meaningful causal hypothesis, but the size of the causal estimate has limited utility. Priorities in such an analysis are to find genetic variants that satisfy the instrumental variable assumptions and to test their associations with the outcome in the largest available dataset that is relevant to the causal question of interest.

In contrast, if investigators seek to estimate the quantitative impact on the outcome of a proposed intervention in the exposure, then further questions become more important, such as how well the genetic variants proxy the specific intervention, whether genetic associations with the exposure are estimated in a relevant population, and whether the relationships between variables are linear and homogeneous in the population. However, causal estimates from Mendelian randomization should always be interpreted with caution (Chapter 6).

Investigators should also give thought to the scope of their analysis. If the aim of the investigation is to understand disease aetiology, then consideration of a limited set of exposures and/or outcomes as main analyses may be justified, whereas if the question relates to public health, then consideration of a broad range of outcomes influenced by an exposure may be worthwhile. At the extreme end of the spectrum is a phenome-wide Mendelian randomization investigation, in which very large numbers of outcomes are considered [Millard et al., 2019]. Such analyses are generally regarded as exploratory or hypothesis-generating, and results are typically treated as provisional until replicated in an independent dataset.

Pre-specifying the primary analyses in a Mendelian randomization investigation is important to address problems of multiple testing, particularly given the large number of analyses that could be performed using available genetic data. Additional analyses, including subgroup analyses and analyses of related outcomes may be presented as supplementary, exploratory or sensitivity analyses. An overly conservative approach to multiple testing may be too strict, given the typically low power of Mendelian randomization studies and the fact that Mendelian randomization often investigates exposure–outcome relationships with prior epidemiological or biological support. As with all epidemiological analyses, it is good practice to avoid selective reporting of statistically significant results (leading to reporting bias) and to describe transparently all analyses performed.

10.2   Data sources

The next fundamental question is which data sources will be used: how many datasets are included in the analysis and whether the analysis is performed using individual-level data or summarized data (Section 2.4).

There are benefits and limitations of both one- and two-sample settings. A one-sample setting allows the investigation to be conducted in a single population sample, meaning that Mendelian randomization and conventional epidemiological findings (for example, from multivariable-adjusted regression) can be compared in the same individuals. In a two-sample setting, the populations from which the two samples were extracted may differ. This is problematic if associations of the genetic variants with the exposure or with variables on pleiotropic pathways differ between the two samples, as this could affect the validity of the instrumental variable assumptions. A particular concern arises if the two samples represent different ethnic groups, as patterns of linkage disequilibrium can differ between populations, meaning that a genetic variant may not be as strongly (or even not at all) associated with the exposure in the outcome dataset. Alternatively, the two samples could differ substantially according to population characteristics such as age, sex, socio-economic background, and so on. Such differences can affect not only the interpretation of causal estimates, but also the validity of causal inferences. For example, genetic variants associated with smoking intensity may be strongly associated with disease outcomes in populations where smoking is common, but not in populations where smoking is rare. One-sample analyses do not suffer from these concerns, nor do they require harmonization of the genetic variants across the datasets (Section 10.4). One- and two-sample investigations also differ in terms of weak instrument bias (Section 8.1). In a two-sample setting without sample overlap, bias due to weak instruments is in the direction of the null, and does not lead to false positive findings.

A related issue is whether the analysis is performed using individual-level data or summarized data. Although the use of summarized data is often synonymous with the two-sample setting, the benefits and limitations for the analysis of the two choices (one- vs two-sample and individual-level vs summarized data) are distinct. Summarized data are often available for larger sample sizes, meaning that power to detect a causal effect is increased. Another advantage of publicly-available summarized data is transparency, as the analysis can be reproduced by a third party with access to the same data. However, access to only summarized data limits the range of analyses that can be performed. Additionally, if published summarized association estimates have already been adjusted for a variable causally downstream of the exposure or outcome, collider bias may be unavoidable (Section 8.5). Individual-level data are required to choose which variables to adjust for when generating summarized data, or to conduct analyses in specific subgroups or strata of the population.

Finally, the choice of dataset should be guided by the motivation of the analysis. If the relevant causal question relates to a particular population, then investigators should choose a dataset to reflect this.

10.3 Selection of genetic variants

The most important decision to be made in designing a Mendelian randomization investigation is which genetic variants to include in the analysis.

10.3.1 Single gene region or polygenic analysis

First, it is necessary to decide whether the analysis is performed using variants from a single gene region, or using variants from multiple regions of the genome (a polygenic analysis). The former has advantages of specificity – if a gene region has a specific biological link with the exposure, then validity of the Mendelian randomization investigation as an assessment of the causal role of that particular exposure is more plausible. However, if only one gene region is included in the analysis, then several robust statistical analysis methods are not possible, as they assume that some but not all variants violate the instrumental variable assumptions. Variants in the same gene region are likely to either all be valid instruments or all invalid. Additionally, when genetic variants are all valid instruments, power is maximized when genetic variants explain the greatest proportion of variance in the exposure – hence a polygenic Mendelian randomization investigation will typically have greater power than one including variants only from a single gene region.

When the analysis is based on a single gene region, it may be that a single variant is included in the analysis. However, if there are multiple variants that explain independent variance in the exposure, then their inclusion will increase power to detect a causal effect, even if the variants are partially correlated (Section 8.10). With summarized data, appropriate methods should be used to account for correlated variants (Section 5.2.6). If variants in a gene region can be thought of as proxies for an intervention that targets the exposure (such as variants in the *HMGCR* gene region for statin drugs), then the analysis has particular relevance for predicting the effect of that intervention.

10.3.2   Biologically- or statistically-driven selection

For a polygenic analysis, there are two main strategies for selecting variants: either a biologically-driven approach or a statistically-driven approach. The two approaches are not mutually exclusive, and the overall decision of which variants to include may comprise elements from both approaches.

A biological approach to the selection of genetic variants would be to include variants from regions that have a biological link to the exposure of interest. For example, several Mendelian randomization investigations for vitamin D have used variants from four gene regions that are biologically implicated in the synthesis or metabolism of vitamin D [Mokry et al., 2015]. However, caution is required as biological understanding is rarely infallible.

A common statistical approach when selecting genetic variants is to include all variants that are associated with the exposure of interest at a given level of statistical significance (typically, a genome-wide significance threshold, such as $p < 5 \times 10^{-8}$). When genome-wide association studies (GWAS) report 'hits' (that is, variants associated with the trait at the given significance threshold), these are often 'pruned' or 'clumped' to near independence using distance-based or correlation-based thresholds (Section 8.10). For example, there may be hundreds of individual variants in one gene region associated with the trait, but these do not represent independent signals. Variants may be pruned to only include one variant in each 500 kilobasepair window (that is, variants must be separated by at least 500 000 basepairs), or variants may only be included that are correlated at $r^2 < 0.01$. If the set of variants is not pruned to near independence, then correlation between the variants may remain, and should be accounted for in a summarized data analysis; even a 500 kilobasepair distance may not be enough to ensure that correlations are close to zero.

If genetic variants are chosen solely based on their association with the exposure without reference to the function of the variants, then researchers should be especially aware about the possibility of variants being pleiotropic. So a more nuanced approach to variant selection would be to start off with a statistical rationale for choosing genetic variants, but then to exclude variants that are known to be pleiotropic or that are associated with variables that represent pleiotropic pathways to the outcome. However, a genetic association with such a variable does not necessarily imply that the instrumental variable assumptions are violated (Figure 3.3).

10.3.3   Dataset for variant selection

Often, variant selection is based on the dataset in which genetic associations with the exposure are estimated. However, this leads to 'winner's curse' – genetic associations tend to be overestimated in the dataset in which they were first discovered (Section 8.4). If genetic variants are selected based on their associations with the exposure in the dataset under analysis, weak instrument bias is exacerbated (in the direction of the observational association in a one-sample setting, and in the direction of the null in a two-sample setting). Bias can be avoided by selecting genetic variants based on a different dataset entirely. This can lead to a 'three-sample' analysis, in which variants are identified in one dataset, and the genetic associations with the exposure and outcome are estimated in separate datasets [Zhao et al., 2019].

10.3.4   Summary of variant selection

To summarize, there is no single correct way to choose which genetic variants to include in an analysis. Causal conclusions will be more reliable when the instrumental variable assumptions are more plausible. Analyses of exposures such as proteins conducted using variants in a coding gene region for the protein (referred to as 'cis-variants'), or otherwise where variants having biological relevance to the exposure can be found, are likely to be more credible. Analyses based on cis-variants only are also likely to be more reliable for assessing the causal role of molecular phenotypes such as gene expression and DNA methylation. However, in many cases (and particularly for multifactorial exposures such as body mass index or blood pressure), it is not possible to find a cis-variant, and so a more agnostic polygenic analysis is necessary. This allows investigators to test for consistency of the causal finding across multiple variants that influence the exposure via different biological pathways. A balance needs to be struck between including fewer variants (and potentially having insufficient power) and including more variants (and potentially including pleiotropic variants).

A practical suggestion for performing a polygenic analysis is to consider both a liberal analysis, including more genetic variants, and a conservative analysis, including fewer variants [Burgess et al., 2015c]. While it is theoretically possible for pleiotropy to lead to a false negative finding, it is generally more likely that pleiotropy will bias estimates away from the null. Hence a null finding in a liberal analysis is more convincing evidence of a true null relationship – there is little evidence for a causal relationship even when potentially pleiotropic genetic variants are included in the analysis. If a non-null causal relationship is indicated in a liberal analysis, the robustness of this finding can be interrogated in further analyses (Figure 10.3).

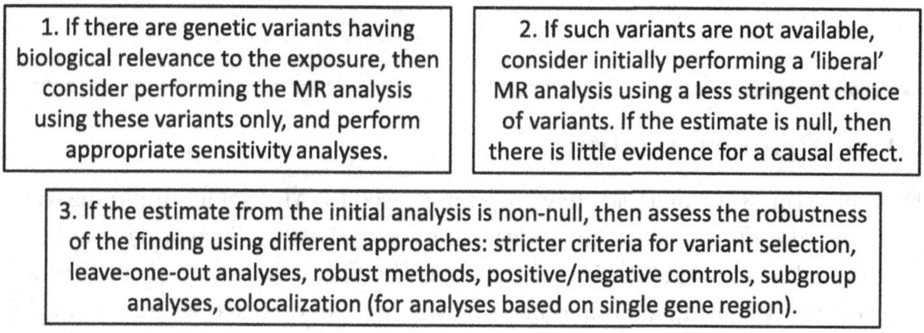

1. If there are genetic variants having biological relevance to the exposure, then consider performing the MR analysis using these variants only, and perform appropriate sensitivity analyses.	2. If such variants are not available, consider initially performing a 'liberal' MR analysis using a less stringent choice of variants. If the estimate is null, then there is little evidence for a causal effect.

3. If the estimate from the initial analysis is non-null, then assess the robustness of the finding using different approaches: stricter criteria for variant selection, leave-one-out analyses, robust methods, positive/negative controls, subgroup analyses, colocalization (for analyses based on single gene region).

FIGURE 10.3
Generic analytic guidelines for Mendelian randomization (MR).

10.4 Variant harmonization

Genetic associations with exposures and outcomes are typically reported per additional copy of a particular allele. Hence, when combining summarized data on genetic associations, it is necessary to ensure that genetic associations are expressed per additional copy of the same allele [Hartwig et al., 2016]. This is particularly important as not all publicly-available data resources are consistent about reporting strand information correctly. For example, if a genetic variant is a biallelic single nucleotide polymorphism (SNP) with alleles A and G on the positive strand, then the corresponding base pairs on the negative strand will be T and C. In this case, one dataset may report the association per additional copy of the A allele, and another per additional copy of the T allele – but the same comparison is being made. Allele and strand information can be double-checked by comparing allele frequency information – if the allele frequencies are similar for the A and T alleles, then the researcher can be more confident that this is a strand mismatch. Additional care should be taken for palindromic variants – if the alleles were A and T (or C and G), then the same alleles would appear on both the positive and negative strands. In such a case, if the allele frequency is close to 50%, it may be necessary to drop the variant from the analysis if it is not possible to verify that the alleles have been correctly orientated. While this is a conservative recommendation, allele alignment problems have led to incorrect results in Mendelian randomization analyses, and retractions and corrections of manuscripts.

10.5 Primary analysis

Different statistical methods have been proposed for Mendelian randomization with individual-level data and with summarized data. Two-stage methods (individual-level data, Section 4.2), such as the two-stage least squares (2SLS) method for a continuous outcome, and the inverse-variance weighted (IVW) method (summarized data, Section 5.2) are the most efficient analysis methods with valid instrumental variables [Wooldridge, 2009a], and so should generally be used as the primary analysis method. The reasoning is the same as for the choice of variants: to first assess evidence for a causal effect in an analysis that assumes all the genetic variants are valid instrumental variables, and then (if a causal effect is evidenced) to interrogate this finding in further analyses. We recommend a multiplicative random-effects model in the IVW method (Section 5.3.1) as this accounts for heterogeneity in the variant-specific causal estimates. Even when investigators have access to individual-level data, calculating summarized data and implementing the IVW method with random-effects is advised to assess robustness to the assumption of balanced pleiotropy.

A scenario that requires a different approach to the primary analysis occurs when there are several related exposures that have shared genetic predictors, meaning that it is difficult to find specific predictors of the individual exposures. In this case, a multivariable Mendelian randomization approach may be the primary analysis strategy (Section 9.1). Both the 2SLS and IVW methods can be adapted to the multivariable setting.

10.6   Robust methods for sensitivity analysis

A robust analysis method is defined as a method that can provide valid causal inferences under weaker assumptions than the standard IVW method. Any polygenic Mendelian randomization investigation that does not perform one or more robust methods may be viewed as somewhat incomplete [Burgess et al., 2017a; Hemani et al., 2018a]. Investigators should consider using multiple methods that make different assumptions about the nature of the underlying pleiotropy (see Chapter 7 for more detail).

While it would be excessive to perform every robust method for Mendelian randomization that has been proposed, investigators should pick a sensible range of methods to assess the sensitivity of their findings. A suggestion is to perform the MR-Egger, weighted median method, and either the mode-based method or contamination mixture method, as these methods require different assumptions to be satisfied for asymptotically consistent estimates. If estimates from all methods are similar, then any causal claim is more credible. However, differences between estimates does not necessarily imply the absence of a causal effect. Different methods will perform better and worse in different scenarios, so critical thought and judgement is required.

We also recommend that a measure of the heterogeneity between variant-specific causal estimates, such as Cochran's Q statistic or the I^2 statistic, is reported as a part of a polygenic Mendelian randomization investigation [Bowden et al., 2018a]. Conclusions are more reliable when multiple genetic variants provide concordant evidence for a causal effect, and particularly when there is no more heterogeneity between the variant-specific causal estimates than expected by chance. Some heterogeneity may be expected even when all genetic variants are valid instruments (Section 5.3). However, causal conclusions are less reliable when there is substantial heterogeneity, especially when there are distinct outliers (which may represent pleiotropic variants) or when evidence for a causal effect depends on one or a small number of variants.

10.7   Other approaches for sensitivity analysis

Sensitivity analysis should not be limited to the application of different statistical methods. This is particularly important for investigations based on a single gene region, as the robust methods discussed above are not applicable in this case. Other approaches for assessing robustness include varying the dataset and choice of genetic variants in the analysis (as in the suggestion of liberal and conservative variant sets in Section 10.3), the use of positive and negative control outcomes, leave-one-out analyses, colocalization, subgroup analyses, and examining associations with potentially pleiotropic variables. We continue to describe each of these in turn.

10.7.1   Positive and negative controls

A positive control outcome is an outcome for which it is already established that the exposure is causal. For example, the outcome of gout may be used as a positive control in a Mendelian randomization investigation for serum uric acid as an exposure, as raised uric acid levels are known to increase risk of gout. Provided that there is sufficient statistical power, then if genetic variants that are associated with serum uric acid are not also associated with risk of gout, then we may question whether the genetic variants are truly able to assess the effect of varying serum uric acid [Palmer et al., 2013]. Conversely, a negative control outcome is an outcome for which it is believed that the exposure cannot be causal. For example, pre-pubertal asthma was used as a negative control outcome in a Mendelian randomization study on the effects of age at puberty on asthma [Minelli et al., 2018]. If a Mendelian randomization investigation suggests that the negative control is caused by the exposure, then violation of the instrumental variable assumptions may be suspected.

10.7.2   Identifying pleiotropic variants and leave-one-out analyses

Leave-one-out analyses (that is, remove one variant from the analysis and re-estimate the causal effect) can be valuable in assessing the reliance of a Mendelian randomization analysis on a particular variant [Corbin et al., 2016]. If there is one genetic variant that is particularly strongly associated with the exposure, then it may dominate the estimate of the causal effect. Investigators should assess the robustness of findings to the removal of such variants. If a causal effect is only evidenced by one variant, then the validity of inference depends only on that variant. If there are many variants in an analysis, leaving one variant out at a time is unlikely to change the estimate substantially, and leaving out subsets of the variants (say, a randomly-chosen 30% at a time [Smith et al., 2014]) may be more appropriate. A further approach for identifying variants to remove from the analysis is Steiger filtering, which removes variants from the analysis if their association with the outcome is stronger than that with the exposure [Hemani et al., 2017b]. It is unlikely that variants could have a stronger association with the outcome than the exposure if the instrumental variable assumptions are satisfied and the genetic association with the outcome is entirely mediated via the exposure.

While removing directly pleiotropic variants from a Mendelian randomization analysis will improve the validity of causal inferences, there is some danger in a *post hoc* or data-driven selection of genetic variants. This is particularly true if the causal effects estimated from many genetic variants are judged to be heterogeneous: the removal of too many variants from the analysis could provide a false impression of agreement amongst the remaining variants, and over-precision in the causal estimate. Removing a variant from the analysis is more justified when a pleiotropic association of the variant has been identified [Cho et al., 2020].

10.7.3 Colocalization

Colocalization assesses whether the same genetic variant (or variants) influences two traits [Hormozdiari et al., 2014; Giambartolomei et al., 2014]. Even if genetic variants in a given gene region are associated with both an exposure and an outcome, this does not imply that the same genetic variants influence both exposure and outcome (meaning there is likely to be a causal pathway including the exposure and outcome). It may be that the two associations are driven by different causal variants, and these variants are correlated due to linkage disequilibrium [Solovieff et al., 2013]. An example of this is the *APOE* gene region, in which genetic variants are associated with both LDL-cholesterol and Alzheimer's disease (Figure 5.2), but LDL-cholesterol does not appear to be a cause of Alzheimer's disease [Benn et al., 2017]. Colocalization can be useful for assessing exposures such as proteins and gene expression, particularly when the Mendelian randomization analysis is based on a single gene region [Zheng et al., 2020]. However, there are several limitations to such an analysis, including whether gene expression is estimated in a relevant tissue. Although colocalization differs from Mendelian randomization in a number of ways, the approach can provide evidence supporting or questioning the evidence at a specific genetic locus for the presence of a biological mechanism linking the exposure and outcome.

10.7.4   Subgroup analyses

A subgroup analysis compares Mendelian randomization estimates estimated in different subgroups of the population for which the genetic variants have different degrees of association with the exposure [van Kippersluis and Rietveld, 2018]. Such an analysis could be performed if there is a subgroup of the population that has reduced or increased levels of the exposure. However, if the subgroup is defined by a collider, then stratification can introduce bias to the analysis (Section 8.5).

10.7.5   Associations with measured covariates

A further possible sensitivity analysis is to check the genetic associations with other variables associated with the outcome, and which are thought not to lie on the causal pathway through the exposure (that is, they are not mediators). Such variables may lie on alternative pleiotropic pathways to the outcome. If the genetic variants are not associated with such variables, then some reassurance can be drawn that the Mendelian randomization assumptions are satisfied. A further possibility in this case is to perform a multivariable Mendelian randomization, including the putative pleiotropic variables as additional exposures in the analysis model [Grant and Burgess, 2020a]. This analysis will estimate the direct effect of the exposure on the outcome keeping these variables constant.

10.8   Data presentation

An attractive feature of Mendelian randomization is that the analysis can be summarized graphically in a transparent way. For example, in a polygenic analysis, a scatter plot of the genetic associations with the outcome against the genetic associations with the exposure reveals much about the analysis – whether different genetic variants provide similar estimates of the causal effect or if there is considerable heterogeneity, and whether the analysis is dominated by a single genetic variant or not. The scatter plot is appealing as it presents the data with no manipulation. Examples of scatter plots illustrating heterogeneity and no heterogeneity in the causal estimates from different variants are shown in Figure 10.4. Alternatives are forest plots, funnel plots, and radial plots – each of these allows heterogeneity in the variant-specific causal estimates to be assessed [Bowden et al., 2018b].

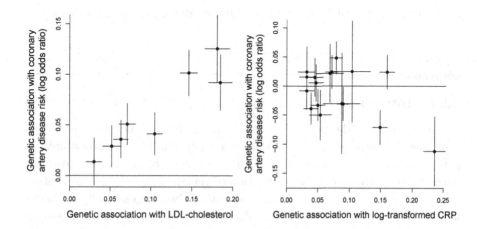

FIGURE 10.4

Scatter plot of genetic associations with the outcome (vertical axis) against genetic associations with the exposure (horizontal axis) for examples illustrating: (left) no heterogeneity in the variant-specific causal estimates (effect of LDL-cholesterol on coronary heart disease risk using eight variants associated with LDL-cholesterol); and (right) heterogeneity in the variant-specific causal estimates (effect of C-reactive protein on coronary heart disease risk using 17 genome-wide significant predictors of C-reactive protein). Lines represent 95% confidence intervals. Taken from Burgess et al. [2018b].

Other important information to report include the R^2 statistic (when the exposure is continuous) and (particularly in a one-sample setting) the F statistic, which is a measure of instrument strength and can be used to judge the extent of weak instrument bias (Section 8.1.2). Investigators can also make some statement about the power of their analysis (Section 8.9). Power calculations are often performed *post hoc*, as sample sizes are rarely determined based on a proposed Mendelian randomization analysis. Power calculations are more meaningful when performed prior to the analysis, and can guide investigators which exposure–outcome pairs to consider, and so focus on analyses that have a better chance of giving meaningful results.

10.9   Interpretation

Finally, we discuss the interpretation of findings from Mendelian randomization investigations. In the first instance, a Mendelian randomization investigation assesses the association of genetic predictors of an exposure with an outcome, or equivalently, the association of genetically-predicted levels of an exposure with an outcome. A statistical test of whether genetically-predicted levels of an exposure are associated with the outcome has an objective interpretation that does not make any untestable assumption. We would encourage primary presentation of results in these terms [Burgess et al., 2020c]. In contrast, making causal inferences from observational data always relies on untestable assumptions. In Mendelian randomization, the assumption is that observed differences in the outcome associated with genetically-predicted levels of the exposure would also be seen if the exposure were intervened on. We recommend that a cautious interpretation should be taken when describing the extent to which a causal effect has been demonstrated by a Mendelian randomization investigation. The appropriate degree of caution will depend on the plausibility of the instrumental variable assumptions, the concordance of estimates from different methods and different analytical approaches, the results from sensitivity and supplementary analyses, and so on.

That said, results from Mendelian randomization investigations have often been shown to qualitatively agree with the results from randomized trials, suggesting that a causal interpretation for Mendelian randomization findings is often reasonable [Haycock et al., 2016]. Mendelian randomization investigations are worthwhile in providing an alternative line of aetiological evidence even though the instrumental variable assumptions can never be proved beyond all doubt [Munafò and Davey, 2018; Lawlor et al.,

2016]. However, quantitative differences between estimates from Mendelian randomization and from trials are likely, particularly as there are differences between how genetic variants influence the exposure as compared to how clinical and pharmaceutical interventions influence the exposure (Chapter 6). Hence, the causal estimate from a Mendelian randomization investigation should not generally be interpreted directly as the expected impact of intervening on the exposure in practice. The estimate from a Mendelian randomization investigation is therefore better interpreted as a test statistic for a causal hypothesis rather than the estimated impact of a well-defined intervention at a specific point in time [Swanson et al., 2017]. But even when a Mendelian randomization investigation is performed primarily to assess the causal role of an exposure, causal estimates can still be useful, for example, to assess heterogeneity in estimates from different variants as a test of instrument validity, or to compare results from different analysis methods as an assessment of robustness. A logical consequence of the 2SLS/IVW method providing the most efficient causal estimate when combining evidence across multiple valid instrumental variables is that, under the same assumptions, the method provides the most powerful test of the presence of a causal effect.

10.10   Summary

Particularly with the advent of summarized data and the two-sample setting, performing a Mendelian randomization analysis has become relatively straightforward. The difficulty is not in performing a Mendelian randomization analysis, but rather in performing a credible analysis.

Overall, the key elements of a Mendelian randomization investigation that we would expect to be present in any manuscript are: i) the motivation for why a Mendelian randomization analysis should be performed and for the scope of the analysis, ii) a clear description and justification of the choice of dataset(s) for the analysis, including why a one- or two-sample approach was chosen for the primary analysis, iii) a clear description and justification of the choice of genetic variants used in the analysis, iv) a discussion, whether statistically or biologically led, of whether the genetic variants are likely to satisfy the instrumental variable assumptions, v) a clear graphical presentation of the data, such as a scatter plot of the genetic associations, and vi) an attempt to test the robustness of the main findings, whether by use of robust methods (for a polygenic analysis) or another approach appropriate to the analysis under consideration. Without these elements, the reader is not able to judge the reliability of a Mendelian randomization investigation.

Part III

Prospects for Mendelian randomization

11

Future directions

In this final chapter, we consider the future of Mendelian randomization within the wider context of epidemiological research. We discuss developments in data availability and methodological practice. These both enable more sophisticated Mendelian randomization analyses and widen the scope for further applications.

11.1 GWAS: large numbers of genetic variants

Genome-wide association studies (GWAS) have driven the rise of Mendelian randomization, by identifying genetic variants that can be used as instrumental variables. They also provide datasets to estimate genetic associations with exposures and outcomes that enable efficient two-sample Mendelian randomization analyses. As the scale and scope of GWAS increase, this will continue to fuel larger and more detailed Mendelian randomization analyses for established risk factors, as well as enable analyses for novel exposures and provide new variants for gene-specific analyses.

11.1.1 Is more variants always better?

While Mendelian randomization analyses based on genetic variants that have demonstrable biological relevance to risk factors are the most reliable, analyses based on large numbers of genetic variants from a GWAS can also provide important evidence to address causal hypotheses. As more genetic variants are discovered that are associated with complex traits, the possibilities for performing Mendelian randomization increase. For risk factors such as blood pressure, several hundred independent associated variants have already been identified in GWAS analyses [Evangelou et al., 2018]. Each additional variant increases the explained proportion of variance in the exposure, potentially increasing the power of a subsequent Mendelian randomization analysis.

However, in including more and more variants, there is likely to be a trade-off between precision and bias. If pleiotropic effects are similar in magnitude for variants having different strengths of association with the exposure, then variants that explain a greater proportion of variance in the exposure are less susceptible to bias due to pleiotropy [Small and Rosenbaum, 2008]. Hence adding progressively more and more variants will add ever decreasing amounts of signal, and proportionally greater amounts of potential noise to the analysis. So while the increasing size of GWAS allows for greater genetic discovery, enabling adequately-powered Mendelian randomization analyses to be performed for more traits, there may come a point at which this provides limited benefit to a polygenic Mendelian randomization analysis for a given trait. Moreover, if the addition of more variants leads to more heterogeneity in the variant-specific estimates, then under a random-effects model the precision of the causal estimate (and hence the power of the analysis) may decrease.

11.1.2   Triangulation of evidence

On the other hand, the availability of large numbers of genetic variants makes robust methods for Mendelian randomization more feasible. In general, we advise caution in the interpretation of findings from a Mendelian randomization investigation with a large number of genetic variants. It is increasingly unlikely that a Mendelian randomization analysis will provide a null result as the sample size increases and more variants are included in the analysis. While this increases power to detect a causal effect, it also increases the possibility of a false positive finding (Type 1 error). This is because as the precision of the estimate increases and its confidence intervals narrow, even a small amount of bias will be enough to result in a non-null estimate. However, several robust methods requires many variants to provide reasonable inferences, and so the availability of larger numbers of genetic variants enables more reliable findings through the principle of triangulation of evidence: evidence for a finding is stronger when the same conclusion is reached by several approaches that make different assumptions [Lawlor et al., 2016].

11.1.3   Subsets and clusters of variants

The increasing number of variants associated with traits provides additional opportunities. In addition to robust methods, which can become increasingly more sophisticated as more data on genetic associations are available, analyses can be performed using subsets of genetic variants that represent specific causal mechanisms. For example, genetic variants that are associated with body mass index (BMI) may influence BMI by various mechanisms, such as suppressing appetite or increasing metabolic rate. If genetic variants can be categorized as associated with one or other of these mechanisms, then separate Mendelian randomization estimates can be obtained using each category of variants [Walter et al., 2015]. Differences in the causal estimates using genetic variants associated with different mechanisms may be informative in understanding disease aetiology, and may highlight specific mechanisms to prioritize for clinical intervention [Burgess et al., 2020b]. Statistical clustering approaches have also been proposed to attempt to search in an agnostic way for subsets of variants with similar variant-specific estimates that may represent distinct causal mechanisms [Foley et al., 2020].

11.2 -omics: Large numbers of risk factors

The term '-omics' covers a broad range of fields of study in cell biology and beyond resulting from developments in high-throughput analytical techniques. Examples of -omics fields include studies of gene expression and methylation (epigenomics), proteins (proteomics), lipids (lipidomics), transcription factors (transcriptomics), and metabolites (metabolomics) [Relton and Davey Smith, 2012]. Relationships between epigenetic markers, proteins, transcription factors and metabolites can be affected by confounding and reverse causation in the same way as relationships between phenotypic exposures and outcomes. Hence such measurements can be used as exposures in Mendelian randomization analyses. As they are more proximal to the genetic code, it is hoped that genetic variants will explain more variance in these -omics measurements than in conventional epidemiological risk factors.

Although -omics data share some common characteristics, each field of study has its own specific challenges for Mendelian randomization investigations. One common characteristic is that measurements may represent a high-dimensional set of related exposure variables with shared genetic predictors. For example, there are often shared predictors of gene expression for neighbouring genes, and the same genetic variants have been shown to predict multiple lipid subtypes. This may necessitate a multivariable Mendelian randomization analysis approach (Section 9.1). Analytic approaches have been developed for combining variable selection and multivariable Mendelian randomization to identify which out of a set of highly correlated traits are causal risk factors for the outcome [Zuber et al., 2020].

11.3   Hypothesis-free: Large numbers of outcomes

In addition to large numbers of risk factors, analyses can be performed for a large number of outcome variables. Investigators can use the same genetic variants in each analysis, testing the association of the variants with each outcome in turn. On the one hand, this enables the broad consequences of intervention on the exposure to be investigated. This is important from a public health perspective, as it may be necessary to balance effects that are in different directions. For example, genetic associations for variants in the *IL1RN* gene region have opposing associations with rheumatoid arthritis and coronary heart disease (Section 5.1). This suggests that interventions that inhibit interleukin-1 reduce the risk of rheumatoid arthritis, but may increase the risk of coronary heart disease [The Interleukin-1 Genetics Consortium, 2015]. A similar balance must be struck for statin drugs, which lower the risk of coronary heart disease, but increase the risk of Type 2 diabetes [Lotta et al., 2016] and possibly haemorrhagic stroke [Sun et al., 2019a]. However, multiple testing is a potential limitation to the interpretation of such analyses. Validation of results in independent datasets is important, particularly for phenome-wide association studies, in which genetic associations with a large number of outcomes are considered in a 'hypothesis-free' way.

11.4   Biobanks: Large numbers of participants

A biobank is a large population-based cross-sectional or longitudinal study. Biobanks are typically designed without a specific research question in mind, but rather gather data on a large number of variables, including phenotypic variables and disease events. Several biobanks (including UK Biobank, FinnGen, and BioBank Japan) have linked genetic data on individuals, facilitating one-sample Mendelian randomization investigations. One particular advantage of biobank data is that it enables non-linear Mendelian randomization analyses, as this requires individual-level data on genetic variants, exposure and outcome in the same individuals (Section 9.3). Another advantage is the possibility to perform subgroup analyses in particular groups of the population, such as sex-specific analyses, or analyses in non-smokers. Analyses can compare estimates for different outcomes obtained in the same dataset, making such comparisons easier to interpret [Allara et al., 2019].

11.5   Clever designs: The role of epidemiologists

There are certainly many advantages of current developments: Mendelian randomization analyses can be performed quickly, easily, and transparently in large data resources. However, it is also increasingly easy to perform a Mendelian randomization analysis without any critical thought. The formula – conduct a genome-wide association study, take all genome-wide significant variants, perform a two-sample analysis – can certainly increase one's publication count. But can such an analysis be considered a contribution to the scientific literature, as it could have been performed already by a machine in a large automated pipeline for large numbers of risk factors and outcomes? [Hemani et al., 2017a]

So we conclude this book by discussing the role of the analyst. We have already stated that we do not believe there is a single 'right way' to perform a Mendelian randomization. While several aspects of the process of Mendelian randomization can be usefully automated, whether by a high-throughput algorithm or a well-meaning human researcher trying to follow best practice, every epidemiological question is different and requires thought as to how to choose the dataset and focus the analysis plan to produce the most reliable inference [Burgess and Davey Smith, 2019]. Further, contextual judgement is required to interpret the findings of an investigation and the extent to which evidence for a causal effect has been demonstrated, particularly when estimates from different methods or analytical approaches give conflicting answers.

There are ways in which unconventional analysis designs can provide additional evidence in a Mendelian randomization investigation. Cross-generational designs using parental and offspring genotypes have been developed that adjust for variables in the offspring generation to infer the effects of parental exposures on offspring outcomes [Evans et al., 2019]. Alternatively, parental disease outcomes have been used to proxy for disease risk in their offspring (genome-wide analysis by proxy) [Liu et al., 2017]. An association between offspring genotype and parental outcome will be weaker than an association between genotype and outcome for the same individual, but if one association is present then the other should be too. This design was originally conceived to maximize case numbers for diseases of old age but has the additional advantage of avoiding selection bias, as it is unlikely that parent's cause of death would influence whether offspring data are available for analysis. Analyses methods have also been proposed to use data on twins, combining the strengths of twin and Mendelian randomization study designs [Minică et al., 2018]. Finally, within-family Mendelian randomization approaches have been developed, which are less susceptible to population stratification as they make comparisons within sibling pairs [Brumpton et al., 2020]. While the trend in Mendelian randomization has been to rely on statistical methodology to provide robust causal inferences, causal research in epidemiology has traditionally relied on design rather than sophisticated statistical methodology [Rubin, 2008]. Combining the approaches requires ingenuity, but can result in additional insights.

Maybe one day machine learning will have cracked how to best design investigations and triangulate evidence from different sources. But for now Mendelian randomization is still a field where clever human analysts still have an edge over machines.

11.6   Conclusion

In conclusion, Mendelian randomization is a powerful, but fallible approach for obtaining causal inferences from observational data. In some cases, it can provide convincing evidence for a causal effect. In other cases, the evidence it provides is valuable, but also far from indisputable. We hope that the material in this book helps you to perform reliable Mendelian randomization investigations and interpret their results honestly, and that their findings advance our knowledge about causal mechanisms relating to disease processes.

Bibliography

Allara, E., Morani, G., Carter, P., et al. 2019. Genetic determinants of lipids and cardiovascular disease outcomes: a wide-angled Mendelian randomization investigation. *Circulation: Genomic and Precision Medicine*, 12(12):e002711. (Cited on page 190.)

Almon, R., Álvarez-Leon, E., Engfeldt, P., Serra-Majem, L., Magnuson, A., and Nilsson, T. 2010. Associations between lactase persistence and the metabolic syndrome in a cross-sectional study in the Canary Islands. *European Journal of Nutrition*, 49(3):141–146. (Cited on page 10.)

Anderson, T. and Rubin, H. 1949. Estimators of the parameters of a single equation in a complete set of stochastic equations. *Annals of Mathematical Statistics*, 21(1):570–582. (Cited on pages 59 and 129.)

Angrist, J., Graddy, K., and Imbens, G. 2000. The interpretation of instrumental variables estimators in simultaneous equations models with an application to the demand for fish. *Review of Economic Studies*, 67(3):499–527. (Cited on pages 61 and 156.)

Angrist, J., Imbens, G., and Rubin, D. 1996. Identification of causal effects using instrumental variables. *Journal of the American Statistical Association*, 91(434):444–455. (Cited on pages 42, 46, and 156.)

Angrist, J. and Pischke, J. 2009a. *Mostly harmless econometrics: an empiricist's companion. Chapter 4: Instrumental variables in action: sometimes you get what you need.* Princeton University Press. (Cited on pages 61, 62, and 146.)

Angrist, J. and Pischke, J. 2009b. *Mostly harmless econometrics: an empiricist's companion. Section 4.6.1: 2SLS mistakes.* Princeton University Press. (Cited on page 137.)

Balke, A. and Pearl, J. 1997. Bounds on treatment effects from studies with imperfect compliance. *Journal of the American Statistical Association*, 92(439):1171–1176. (Cited on page 146.)

Baum, C., Schaffer, M., and Stillman, S. 2003. Instrumental variables and GMM: Estimation and testing. *Stata Journal*, 3(1):1–31. (Cited on page 64.)

Bech, B., Autrup, H., Nohr, E., Henriksen, T., and Olsen, J. 2006. Stillbirth and slow metabolizers of caffeine: comparison by genotypes. *International Journal of Epidemiology*, 35(4):948–953. (Cited on page 10.)

Beer, N., Tribble, N., McCulloch, L., et al. 2009. The P446L variant in *GCKR* associated with fasting plasma glucose and triglyceride levels exerts its effect through increased glucokinase activity in liver. *Human Molecular Genetics*, 18(21):4081–4088. (Cited on page 94.)

Bekker, P. 1994. Alternative approximations to the distributions of instrumental variable estimators. *Econometrica: Journal of the Econometric Society*, 62(3):657–681. (Cited on page 146.)

Benn, M., Nordestgaard, B. G., Frikke-Schmidt, R., and Tybjærg-Hansen, A. 2017. Low LDL cholesterol, *PCSK9* and *HMGCR* genetic variation, and risk of Alzheimer's disease and Parkinson's disease: Mendelian randomisation study. *British Medical Journal*, 357:j1648. (Cited on page 179.)

Beral, V., Banks, E., Bull D., Reeves, G. (Million Women Study Collaborators) 2003. Breast cancer and hormone-replacement therapy in the Million Women Study. *The Lancet*, 362(9382):419–427. (Cited on page 5.)

Berzuini, C., Guo, H., Burgess, S., and Bernardinelli, L. 2020. A Bayesian approach to mendelian randomization with multiple pleiotropic variants. *Biostatistics*, 21(1):86–101. (Cited on page 116.)

Bochud, M., Chiolero, A., Elston, R., and Paccaud, F. 2008. A cautionary note on the use of Mendelian randomization to infer causation in observational epidemiology. *International Journal of Epidemiology*, 37(2):414–416. (Cited on page 36.)

Bochud, M. and Rousson, V. 2010. Usefulness of Mendelian randomization in observational epidemiology. *International Journal of Environmental Research and Public Health*, 7(3):711–728. (Cited on page 9.)

Borenstein, M., Hedges, L., Higgins, J., and Rothstein, H. 2009. *Introduction to meta-analysis. Chapter 34: Generality of the basic inverse-variance method.* Wiley. (Cited on page 70.)

Bound, J., Jaeger, D., and Baker, R. 1995. Problems with instrumental variables estimation when the correlation between the instruments and the endogenous explanatory variable is weak. *Journal of the American Statistical Association*, 90(430):443–450. (Cited on page 123.)

Bowden, J., Davey Smith, G., and Burgess, S. 2015. Mendelian randomization with invalid instruments: effect estimation and bias detection through Egger regression. *International Journal of Epidemiology*, 44(2):512–525. (Cited on pages 105 and 111.)

Bowden, J., Davey Smith, G., Haycock, P. C., and Burgess, S. 2016. Consistent estimation in Mendelian randomization with some invalid instruments using a weighted median estimator. *Genetic Epidemiology*, 40(4):304–314. (Cited on pages 104 and 105.)

Bowden, J., Del Greco, F., Minelli, C., et al. 2019. Improving the accuracy of two-sample summary data Mendelian randomization: moving beyond the NOME assumption. *International Journal of Epidemiology*, 48(3):728–742. (Cited on page 72.)

Bowden, J., Hemani, G., and Davey Smith, G. 2018a. Detecting individual and global horizontal pleiotropy in Mendelian randomization – a job for the humble heterogeneity statistic? *American Journal of Epidemiology*, 187(12):2681–2685. (Cited on page 177.)

Bowden, J., Spiller, W., Del Greco M, F., et al. 2018b. Improving the visualization, interpretation and analysis of two-sample summary data Mendelian randomization via the Radial plot and Radial regression. *International Journal of Epidemiology*, 47(4):1264–1278. (Cited on pages 74 and 180.)

Bowden, J. and Vansteelandt, S. 2011. Mendelian randomisation analysis of case-control data using structural mean models. *Statistics in Medicine*, 30(6):678–694. (Cited on pages 56 and 57.)

Brumpton, B., Sanderson, E., Heilbron, K., et al. 2020. Avoiding dynastic, assortative mating, and population stratification biases in Mendelian randomization through within-family analyses. *Nature Communications*, 11:3519. (Cited on page 192.)

Buonaccorsi, J. 2005. *Encyclopedia of Biostatistics*, chapter Fieller's theorem, pages 1951–1952. Wiley. (Cited on page 59.)

Burgess, S. 2014. Sample size and power calculations in Mendelian randomization with a single instrumental variable and a binary outcome. *International Journal of Epidemiology*, 43(3):922–929. (Cited on page 141.)

Burgess, S. 2015. Commentary: Consistency and collapsibility: are they crucial for instrumental variable analysis with a survival outcome in Mendelian randomization? *Epidemiology*, 26(3):411–413. (Cited on page 140.)

Burgess, S. 2017. Estimating and contextualizing the attenuation of odds ratios due to non-collapsibility. *Communications in Statistics – Theory and Methods*, 46(2):786–804. (Cited on pages 50 and 139.)

Burgess, S., Bowden, J., Dudbridge, F., and Thompson, S. G. 2016a. Robust instrumental variable methods using multiple candidate instruments with application to Mendelian randomization. *arXiv*, 1606.03729. (Cited on page 111.)

Burgess, S., Bowden, J., Fall, T., Ingelsson, E., and Thompson, S. G. 2017a. Sensitivity analyses for robust causal inference from Mendelian randomization analyses with multiple genetic variants. *Epidemiology*, 28(1):30–42. (Cited on pages 74 and 177.)

Burgess, S., Butterworth, A. S., and Thompson, S. G. 2013. Mendelian randomization analysis with multiple genetic variants using summarized data. *Genetic Epidemiology*, 37(7):658–665. (Cited on pages 25 and 105.)

Burgess, S. and CCGC (CHD CRP Genetics Collaboration) 2013. Identifying the odds ratio estimated by a two-stage instrumental variable analysis with a logistic regression model. *Statistics in Medicine*, 32(27):4726–4747. (Cited on pages 50 and 138.)

Burgess, S., Daniel, R., Butterworth, A., Thompson, S., and EPIC-InterAct Consortium 2015a. Network Mendelian randomization: extending instrumental variable techniques. *International Journal of Epidemiology*, 44(2):484–495. (Cited on pages 154 and 164.)

Burgess, S. and Davey Smith, G. 2017. Mendelian randomization implicates high-density lipoprotein cholesterol–associated mechanisms in etiology of age-related macular degeneration. *Ophthalmology*, 124(8):1165–1174. (Cited on pages 10 and 103.)

Burgess, S. and Davey Smith, G. 2019. How humans can contribute to Mendelian randomization analyses. *International Journal of Epidemiology*, 48(3):661–664. (Cited on page 191.)

Burgess, S., Davey Smith, G., Davies, N. M., et al. 2020a. Guidelines for performing Mendelian randomization investigations. *Wellcome Open Research*, 4:186. (Cited on page 167.)

Burgess, S., Davies, N. M., and Thompson, S. G. 2016b. Bias due to participant overlap in two-sample Mendelian randomization. *Genetic Epidemiology*, 40(7):597–608. (Cited on pages 132 and 133.)

Burgess, S., Davies, N. M., Thompson, S. G., and EPIC-InterAct Consortium 2014a. Instrumental variable analysis with a nonlinear exposure–outcome relationship. *Epidemiology*, 25(6):877–885. (Cited on pages 53, 157, and 158.)

Burgess, S., Dudbridge, F., and Thompson, S. G. 2015b. Re: "Multivariable Mendelian randomization: the use of pleiotropic genetic variants to estimate causal effects". *American Journal of Epidemiology*, 181(4):290–291. (Cited on page 151.)

Burgess, S., Dudbridge, F., and Thompson, S. G. 2016c. Combining information on multiple instrumental variables in Mendelian randomization: comparison of allele score and summarized data methods. *Statistics in Medicine*, 35(11):1880–1906. (Cited on page 71.)

Burgess, S., Ference, B. A., Staley, J. R., et al. 2018a. Association of *LPA* variants with risk of coronary disease and the implications for lipoprotein(a)-lowering therapies: a Mendelian randomization analysis. *JAMA Cardiology*, 3(7):619–627. (Cited on pages 89, 91, and 92.)

Burgess, S., Foley, C. N., Allara, E., Staley, J. R., and Howson, J. M. 2020b. A robust and efficient method for Mendelian randomization with hundreds of genetic variants. *Nature Communications*, 11:376. (Cited on pages 105, 115, 118, and 189.)

Burgess, S., Freitag, D. F., Khan, H., Gorman, D. N., and Thompson, S. G. 2014b. Using multivariable Mendelian randomization to disentangle the causal effects of lipid fractions. *PLOS One*, 9(10):e108891. (Cited on page 149.)

Burgess, S., Granell, R., Palmer, T., Didelez, V., and Sterne, J. 2014c. Lack of identification in semi-parametric instrumental variable models with binary outcomes. *American Journal of Epidemiology*, 180(1):111–119. (Cited on page 147.)

Burgess, S. and Labrecque, J. A. 2018. Mendelian randomization with a binary exposure variable: interpretation and presentation of causal estimates. *European Journal of Epidemiology*, 33(10):947–952. (Cited on pages 143 and 145.)

Burgess, S., O'Donnell, C. J., and Gill, D. 2020c. Expressing results from a Mendelian randomization analysis: separating results from inferences. *JAMA Cardiology*. (Cited on page 182.)

Burgess, S., Scott, R., Timpson, N., Davey Smith, G., Thompson, S. G., and EPIC-InterAct Consortium 2015c. Using published data in Mendelian randomization: a blueprint for efficient identification of causal risk factors. *European Journal of Epidemiology*, 30(7):543–552. (Cited on pages 25 and 175.)

Burgess, S., Thompson, D. J., Rees, J. M., Day, F. R., Perry, J. R., and Ong, K. K. 2017b. Dissecting causal pathways using Mendelian randomization with summarized genetic data: application to age at menarche and risk of breast cancer. *Genetics*, 207:481–487. (Cited on pages 151, 152, and 153.)

Burgess, S. and Thompson, S. G. 2011. Bias in causal estimates from Mendelian randomization studies with weak instruments. *Statistics in Medicine*, 30(11):1312–1323. (Cited on pages 121, 123, and 126.)

Burgess, S. and Thompson, S. G. 2012. Improvement of bias and coverage in instrumental variable analysis with weak instruments for continuous and binary outcomes. *Statistics in Medicine*, 31(15):1582–1600. (Cited on pages 63 and 139.)

Burgess, S. and Thompson, S. G. 2013. Use of allele scores as instrumental variables for Mendelian randomization. *International Journal of Epidemiology*, 42(4):1134–1144. (Cited on pages 130 and 131.)

Burgess, S. and Thompson, S. G. 2015. Multivariable Mendelian randomization: the use of pleiotropic genetic variants to estimate causal effects. *American Journal of Epidemiology*, 181(4):251–260. (Cited on page 149.)

Burgess, S. and Thompson, S. G. 2017. Interpreting findings from Mendelian randomization using the MR-Egger method. *European Journal of Epidemiology*, 32(5):377–389. (Cited on pages 112, 113, and 114.)

Burgess, S., Thompson, S. G., and CRP CHD Genetics Collaboration 2010. Bayesian methods for meta-analysis of causal relationships estimated using genetic instrumental variables. *Statistics in Medicine*, 29(12):1298–1311. (Cited on page 146.)

Burgess, S., Thompson, S. G., and CRP CHD Genetics Collaboration 2011. Avoiding bias from weak instruments in Mendelian randomization studies. *International Journal of Epidemiology*, 40(3):755–764. (Cited on pages 126 and 130.)

Burgess, S., Zuber, V., Gkatzionis, A., and Foley, C. N. 2018b. Modal-based estimation via heterogeneity-penalized weighting: model averaging for consistent and efficient estimation in Mendelian randomization when a plurality of candidate instruments are valid. *International Journal of Epidemiology*, 47(4):1242–1254. (Cited on page 181.)

Burgess, S., Zuber, V., Valdes-Marquez, E., Sun, B. B., and Hopewell, J. C. 2017c. Mendelian randomization with fine-mapped genetic data: Choosing from large numbers of correlated instrumental variables. *Genetic Epidemiology*, 41(8):714–725. (Cited on pages 73, 142, and 143.)

Cai, B., Small, D., and Ten Have, T. 2011. Two-stage instrumental variable methods for estimating the causal odds ratio: Analysis of bias. *Statistics in Medicine*, 30(15):1809–1824. (Cited on page 63.)

Carreras-Torres, R., Johansson, M., Haycock, P. C., et al. 2018. Role of obesity in smoking behaviour: Mendelian randomisation study in UK Biobank. *British Medical Journal*, 361:k1767. (Cited on page 165.)

Carter, A. R., Borges, M.-C., Benn, M., et al. 2019a. Combined association of body mass index and alcohol consumption with biomarkers for liver injury and incidence of liver disease: a Mendelian randomization study. *JAMA Network Open*, 2(3):e190305. (Cited on page 162.)

Carter, A. R., Sanderson, E., Hammerton, G., et al. 2019b. Mendelian randomisation for mediation analysis: current methods and challenges for implementation. *bioRxiv*, 835819. (Cited on page 154.)

Casas, J., Bautista, L., Smeeth, L., Sharma, P., and Hingorani, A. 2005. Homocysteine and stroke: evidence on a causal link from Mendelian randomisation. *The Lancet*, 365(9455):224–232. (Cited on page 10.)

CCGC (CRP CHD Genetics Collaboration) 2011. Association between C reactive protein and coronary heart disease: Mendelian randomisation analysis based on individual participant data. *British Medical Journal*, 342:d548. (Cited on page 85.)

Chen, L., Davey Smith, G., Harbord, R., and Lewis, S. 2008. Alcohol intake and blood pressure: a systematic review implementing a Mendelian randomization approach. *PLoS Medicine*, 5(3):e52. (Cited on page 10.)

Cheung, B., Lauder, I., Lau, C., and Kumana, C. 2004. Meta-analysis of large randomized controlled trials to evaluate the impact of statins on cardiovascular outcomes. *British Journal of Clinical Pharmacology*, 57(5):640–651. (Cited on page 87.)

Cho, Y., Haycock, P. C., Sanderson, E., et al. 2020. Exploiting horizontal pleiotropy to search for causal pathways within a Mendelian randomization framework. *Nature Communications*, 11:1010. (Cited on page 179.)

Cho, Y., Shin, S.-Y., Won, S., Relton, C. L., Davey Smith, G., and Shin, M.-J. 2015. Alcohol intake and cardiovascular risk factors: A Mendelian randomisation study. *Scientific Reports*, 5:18422. (Cited on page 135.)

Cholesterol Treatment Trialists' Collaboration 2005. Efficacy and safety of cholesterol-lowering treatment: prospective meta-analysis of data from 90 056 participants in 14 randomised trials of statins. *The Lancet*, 366(9493):1267–1278. (Cited on page 102.)

Christenfeld, N., Sloan, R., Carroll, D., and Greenland, S. 2004. Risk factors, confounding, and the illusion of statistical control. *Psychosomatic Medicine*, 66(6):868–875. (Cited on page 16.)

Clarke, P. S. and Windmeijer, F. 2012. Instrumental variable estimators for binary outcomes. *Journal of the American Statistical Association*, 107(500):1638–1652. (Cited on pages 42 and 147.)

Clarke, R., Peden, J., Hopewell, J., et al. 2009. Genetic variants associated with Lp(a) lipoprotein level and coronary disease. *New England Journal of Medicine*, 361(26):2518–2528. (Cited on pages 10 and 89.)

Cohen, J., Boerwinkle, E., Mosley Jr, T., and Hobbs, H. 2006. Sequence variations in *PCSK9*, low LDL, and protection against coronary heart disease. *New England Journal of Medicine*, 354(12):1264–1272. (Cited on page 94.)

Cole, S. R., Platt, R. W., Schisterman, E. F., et al. 2010. Illustrating bias due to conditioning on a collider. *International Journal of Epidemiology*, 39(2):417–420. (Cited on page 134.)

Collins, R., Armitage, J., Parish, S., Sleight, P., Peto, R. (Heart Protection Study Collaborative Group) 2002. MRC/BHF Heart Protection Study of antioxidant vitamin supplementation in 20536 high-risk individuals: a randomised placebo-controlled trial. *The Lancet*, 360(9326):23–33. (Cited on page 4.)

Corbin, L. J., Richmond, R. C., Wade, K. H., et al. 2016. Body mass index as a modifiable risk factor for type 2 diabetes: Refining and understanding causal estimates using Mendelian randomisation. *Diabetes*, 65(10):3002–3007. (Cited on pages 76 and 178.)

Cox, D. 1958. *Planning of experiments. Section 2: Some key assumptions.* Wiley. (Cited on page 48.)

Danesh, J. and Pepys, M. 2009. C-reactive protein and coronary disease: is there a causal link? *Circulation*, 120(21):2036–2039. (Cited on page 7.)

Darwin, C. 1871. *The descent of man and selection in relation to sex.* Murray, London. (Cited on page 5.)

Dastani, Z., Hivert, M.-F., Timpson, N., et al. 2012. Novel loci for adiponectin levels and their influence on type 2 diabetes and metabolic traits: A multi-ethnic meta-analysis of 45,891 individuals. *PLOS Genetics*, 8(3):e1002607. (Cited on page 71.)

Davey Smith, G. 2006. Randomised by (your) god: robust inference from an observational study design. *Journal of Epidemiology and Community Health*, 60(5):382–388. (Cited on page 84.)

Davey Smith, G. 2011. Use of genetic markers and gene-diet interactions for interrogating population-level causal influences of diet on health. *Genes & Nutrition*, 6(1):27–43. (Cited on page 85.)

Davey Smith, G. and Ebrahim, S. 2003. 'Mendelian randomization': can genetic epidemiology contribute to understanding environmental determinants of disease? *International Journal of Epidemiology*, 32(1):1–22. (Cited on pages 4, 5, and 20.)

Davey Smith, G. and Ebrahim, S. 2004. Mendelian randomization: prospects, potentials, and limitations. *International Journal of Epidemiology*, 33(1):30–42. (Cited on page 24.)

Davey Smith, G., Lawlor, D., Harbord, R., Timpson, N., Day, I., and Ebrahim, S. 2007. Clustered environments and randomized genes: a fundamental distinction between conventional and genetic epidemiology. *PLoS Medicine*, 4(12):e352. (Cited on page 18.)

Davies, N., von Hinke Kessler Scholder, S., Farbmacher, H., Burgess, S., Windmeijer, F., and Davey Smith, G. 2015. The many weak instrument problem and Mendelian randomization. *Statistics in Medicine*, 34(3):454–468. (Cited on page 146.)

Davignon, J. and Laaksonen, R. 1999. Low-density lipoprotein-independent effects of statins. *Current Opinion in Lipidology*, 10(6):543–559. (Cited on page 89.)

Dawid, A. 2000. Causal inference without counterfactuals. *Journal of the American Statistical Association*, 95(450):407–424. (Cited on page 28.)

Dawid, A. 2002. Influence diagrams for causal modelling and inference. *International Statistical Review*, 70(2):161–189. (Cited on page 41.)

Debat, V. and David, P. 2001. Mapping phenotypes: canalization, plasticity and developmental stability. *Trends in Ecology & Evolution*, 16(10):555–561. (Cited on page 35.)

Dekkers, O., von Elm, E., Algra, A., Romijn, J., and Vandenbroucke, J. 2010. How to assess the external validity of therapeutic trials: a conceptual approach. *International Journal of Epidemiology*, 39(1):89–94. (Cited on page 92.)

Didelez, V., Meng, S., and Sheehan, N. 2010. Assumptions of IV methods for observational epidemiology. *Statistical Science*, 25(1):22–40. (Cited on pages 41, 53, and 56.)

Didelez, V. and Sheehan, N. 2007. Mendelian randomization as an instrumental variable approach to causal inference. *Statistical Methods in Medical Research*, 16(4):309–330. (Cited on pages 38, 41, 48, 57, and 170.)

Ding, E., Song, Y., Manson, J., et al. 2009. Sex hormone-binding globulin and risk of type 2 diabetes in women and men. *New England Journal of Medicine*, 361(12):1152–1163. (Cited on page 10.)

Do, R., Willer, C. J., Schmidt, E. M., et al. 2013. Common variants associated with plasma triglycerides and risk for coronary artery disease. *Nature Genetics*, 45:1345–1352. (Cited on page 102.)

Ducharme, G. and LePage, Y. 1986. Testing collapsibility in contingency tables. *Journal of the Royal Statistical Society: Series B (Methodological)*, 48(2):197–205. (Cited on page 138.)

Ebrahim, S. and Davey Smith, G. 2008. Mendelian randomization: can genetic epidemiology help redress the failures of observational epidemiology? *Human Genetics*, 123(1):15–33. (Cited on pages 39 and 60.)

Ehret, G., Munroe, P., Rice, K., et al. (The International Consortium for Blood Pressure Genome-Wide Association Studies) 2011. Genetic variants in novel pathways influence blood pressure and cardiovascular disease risk. *Nature*, 478:103–109. (Cited on page 89.)

Elliott, P., Chambers, J., Zhang, W., et al. 2009. Genetic loci associated with C-reactive protein levels and risk of coronary heart disease. *Journal of the American Medical Association*, 302(1):37–48. (Cited on page 85.)

Eppinga, R. N., Hagemeijer, Y., Burgess, S., et al. 2016. Identification of genomic loci associated with resting heart rate and shared genetic predictors with all-cause mortality. *Nature Genetics*, 48:1557–1563. (Cited on page 10.)

Evangelou, E., Warren, H. R., Mosen-Ansorena, D., et al. 2018. Genetic analysis of over one million people identifies 535 novel loci for blood pressure. *Nature Genetics*, 50:1412–1425. (Cited on page 187.)

Evans, D. M., Moen, G.-H., Hwang, L.-D., Lawlor, D. A., and Warrington, N. M. 2019. Elucidating the role of maternal environmental exposures on offspring health and disease using two-sample Mendelian randomization. *International Journal of Epidemiology*, 48(3):861–875. (Cited on page 191.)

Ference, B. A., Majeed, F., Penumetcha, R., Flack, J. M., and Brook, R. D. 2015. Effect of naturally random allocation to lower low-density lipoprotein cholesterol on the risk of coronary heart disease mediated by polymorphisms in *NPC1L1*, *HMGCR*, or both: a 2 × 2 factorial Mendelian randomization study. *Journal of the American College of Cardiology*, 65(15):1552–1561. (Cited on page 162.)

Ference, B. A., Yoo, W., Alesh, I., et al. 2012. Effect of long-term exposure to lower low-density lipoprotein cholesterol beginning early in life on the risk of coronary heart disease: a Mendelian randomization analysis. *Journal of the American College of Cardiology*, 60(25):2631–2639. (Cited on page 84.)

Fieller, E. 1954. Some problems in interval estimation. *Journal of the Royal Statistical Society: Series B (Statistical Methodology)*, 16(2):175–185. (Cited on page 58.)

Fischer-Lapp, K. and Goetghebeur, E. 1999. Practical properties of some structural mean analyses of the effect of compliance in randomized trials. *Controlled Clinical Trials*, 20(6):531–546. (Cited on page 147.)

Fisher, R. 1918. The correlation between relatives on the supposition of Mendelian inheritance. *Transactions of the Royal Society of Edinburgh*, 52(2):399–433. (Cited on page 5.)

Foley, C. N., Kirk, P. D., and Burgess, S. 2020. MR-Clust: Clustering of genetic variants in Mendelian randomization with similar causal estimates. *Bioinformatics*. (Cited on page 189.)

Foster, E. 1997. Instrumental variables for logistic regression: an illustration. *Social Science Research*, 26(4):487–504. (Cited on pages 62 and 147.)

Frost, C. and Thompson, S. G. 2000. Correcting for regression dilution bias: comparison of methods for a single predictor variable. *Journal of the Royal Statistical Society: Series A (Statistics in Society)*, 163(2):173–189. (Cited on page 20.)

Gage, S. H., Jones, H. J., Burgess, S., et al. 2017. Assessing causality in associations between cannabis use and schizophrenia risk: a two-sample Mendelian randomization study. *Psychological Medicine*, 47(5):971–980. (Cited on pages 10 and 144.)

Gale, C. R. and Martyn, C. N. 1995. Migrant studies in multiple sclerosis. *Progress in Neurobiology*, 47(4-5):425–448. (Cited on page 84.)

Giambartolomei, C., Vukcevic, D., Schadt, E. E., et al. 2014. Bayesian test for colocalisation between pairs of genetic association studies using summary statistics. *PLOS Genetics*, 10(5):e1004383. (Cited on page 179.)

Gill, D., Georgakis, M. K., Zuber, V., et al. 2020. Genetically predicted midlife blood pressure and coronary artery disease risk: Mendelian randomization analysis. *Journal of the American Heart Association*, 9(14):e016773. (Cited on page 140.)

Gkatzionis, A. and Burgess, S. 2019. Contextualizing selection bias in Mendelian randomization: how bad is it likely to be? *International Journal of Epidemiology*, 48(3):691–701. (Cited on page 135.)

Gkatzionis, A., Burgess, S., Conti, D., and Newcombe, P. J. 2019. Bayesian variable selection with a pleiotropic loss function in Mendelian randomization. *bioRxiv*, 593863. (Cited on page 143.)

Glymour, M., Tchetgen Tchetgen, E., and Robins, J. 2012. Credible Mendelian randomization studies: approaches for evaluating the instrumental variable assumptions. *American Journal of Epidemiology*, 175(4):332–339. (Cited on pages 38 and 95.)

Grant, A. J. and Burgess, S. 2020a. An efficient and robust approach to Mendelian randomization with measured pleiotropic effects in a high-dimensional setting. *Biostatistics*. (Cited on pages 152 and 180.)

Grant, A. J. and Burgess, S. 2020b. Pleiotropy robust methods for multivariable Mendelian randomization. *arXiv*, 2008.11997. (Cited on page 151.)

Greco, M., Minelli, C., Sheehan, N. A., and Thompson, J. R. 2015. Detecting pleiotropy in Mendelian randomisation studies with summary data and a continuous outcome. *Statistics in Medicine*, 34(21):2926–2940. (Cited on page 74.)

Greenland, S. 2000a. An introduction to instrumental variables for epidemiologists. *International Journal of Epidemiology*, 29(4):722–729. (Cited on pages 14 and 31.)

Greenland, S. 2000b. Causal analysis in the health sciences. *Journal of the American Statistical Association*, 95(449):286–289. (Cited on page 28.)

Greenland, S. and Robins, J. 1986. Identifiability, exchangeability, and epidemiological confounding. *International Journal of Epidemiology*, 15(3):413–419. (Cited on pages 16, 29, and 32.)

Greenland, S., Robins, J., and Pearl, J. 1999. Confounding and collapsibility in causal inference. *Statistical Science*, 14(1):29–46. (Cited on page 138.)

Gregson, J. M., Freitag, D. F., Surendran, P., et al. 2017. Genetic invalidation of Lp-PLA$_2$ as a therapeutic target: Large-scale study of five functional Lp-PLA$_2$-lowering alleles. *European Journal of Preventive Cardiology*, 24(5):492–504. (Cited on pages 44 and 45.)

Guo, Q., Burgess, S., Turman, C., et al. 2017. Body mass index and breast cancer survival: a Mendelian randomization analysis. *International Journal of Epidemiology*, 46(6):1814–1822. (Cited on page 10.)

Guo, Z., Kang, H., Tony Cai, T., and Small, D. S. 2018. Confidence intervals for causal effects with invalid instruments by using two-stage hard thresholding with voting. *Journal of the Royal Statistical Society: Series B (Statistical Methodology)*, 80(4):793–815. (Cited on page 107.)

Hahn, J., Hausman, J., and Kuersteiner, G. 2004. Estimation with weak instruments: accuracy of higher-order bias and MSE approximations. *Econometrics Journal*, 7(1):272–306. (Cited on page 146.)

Hansen, L. 1982. Large sample properties of generalized method of moments estimators. *Econometrica: Journal of the Econometric Society*, 50(4):1029–1054. (Cited on page 147.)

Hartwig, F. P., Davey Smith, G., and Bowden, J. 2017. Robust inference in summary data Mendelian randomisation via the zero modal pleiotropy assumption. *International Journal of Epidemiology*, 46(6):1985–1998. (Cited on pages 105 and 107.)

Hartwig, F. P. and Davies, N. M. 2016. Why internal weights should be avoided (not only) in MR-Egger regression. *International Journal of Epidemiology*, 45:1676–1678. (Cited on page 129.)

Hartwig, F. P., Davies, N. M., Hemani, G., and Davey Smith, G. 2016. Two-sample Mendelian randomization: avoiding the downsides of a powerful, widely applicable but potentially fallible technique. *International Journal of Epidemiology*, 45(6):1717–1726. (Cited on page 175.)

Hayashi, F. 2000. *Econometrics*. Princeton University Press. (Cited on page 146.)

Haycock, P. C., Burgess, S., Wade, K. H., Bowden, J., Relton, C., and Davey Smith, G. 2016. Best (but oft-forgotten) practices: the design, analysis, and interpretation of Mendelian randomization studies. *The American Journal of Clinical Nutrition*, 103(4):965–978. (Cited on page 182.)

Hemani, G., Bowden, J., and Davey Smith, G. 2018a. Evaluating the potential role of pleiotropy in Mendelian randomization studies. *Human Molecular Genetics*, 27(R2):R195–R208. (Cited on page 177.)

Hemani, G., Bowden, J., Haycock, P. C., et al. 2017a. Automating mendelian randomization through machine learning to construct a putative causal map of the human phenome. *bioRxiv*, 173682. (Cited on page 191.)

Hemani, G., Tilling, K., and Davey Smith, G. 2017b. Orienting the causal relationship between imprecisely measured traits using GWAS summary data. *PLOS Genetics*, 13(11):e1007081. (Cited on page 179.)

Hemani, G., Zheng, J., Elsworth, B., et al. 2018b. The MR-Base platform supports systematic causal inference across the human phenome. *eLife*, 7:e34408. (Cited on page 79.)

Hennekens, C., Buring, J., Manson, J., et al. 1996. Lack of effect of long-term supplementation with beta carotene on the incidence of malignant neoplasms and cardiovascular disease. *New England Journal of Medicine*, 334(18):1145–1149. (Cited on page 4.)

Hernán, M., Hernández-Díaz, S., and Robins, J. 2004. A structural approach to selection bias. *Epidemiology*, 15(5):615–625. (Cited on page 135.)

Hernán, M. and Robins, J. 2006. Instruments for causal inference: an epidemiologist's dream? *Epidemiology*, 17(4):360–372. (Cited on pages 17, 36, and 42.)

Hernán, M. A. 2010. The hazards of hazard ratios. *Epidemiology*, 21(1):13–15. (Cited on page 140.)

Higgins, J., Thompson, S., Deeks, J., and Altman, D. 2003. Measuring inconsistency in meta-analyses. *British Medical Journal*, 327(7414):557–560. (Cited on page 76.)

Hill, A. B. 1965. The environment and disease: association or causation? *Proceedings of the Royal Society of Medicine*, 58(5):295–300. (Cited on page 39.)

Holland, P. 1986. Statistics and causal inference. *Journal of the American Statistical Association*, 81(396):945–960. (Cited on pages 27 and 28.)

Holmes, M. V., Ala-Korpela, M., and Davey Smith, G. 2017. Mendelian randomization in cardiometabolic disease: challenges in evaluating causality. *Nature Reviews Cardiology*, 14(10):577–590. (Cited on page 139.)

Hooper, L., Ness, A., and Davey Smith, G. 2001. Antioxidant strategy for cardiovascular diseases. *The Lancet*, 357(9269):1705–1706. (Cited on page 4.)

Hormozdiari, F., Kostem, E., Kang, E. Y., Pasaniuc, B., and Eskin, E. 2014. Identifying causal variants at loci with multiple signals of association. *Genetics*, 198(2):497–508. (Cited on page 179.)

Hughes, R. A., Davies, N. M., Davey Smith, G., and Tilling, K. 2019. Selection bias when estimating average treatment effects using one-sample instrumental variable analysis. *Epidemiology*, 30(3):350–357. (Cited on page 135.)

Jiang, L., Oualkacha, K., Didelez, V., et al. 2019. Constrained instruments and their application to Mendelian randomization with pleiotropy. *Genetic Epidemiology*, 43(4):373–401. (Cited on page 117.)

Johnson, T. 2013. Efficient calculation for multi-SNP genetic risk scores. Technical report, The Comprehensive R Archive Network. Available at https://github.com/cran/gtx/blob/master/inst/doc/ashg2012.pdf [last accessed 2020/6/17]. (Cited on page 71.)

Johnston, K., Gustafson, P., Levy, A., and Grootendorst, P. 2008. Use of instrumental variables in the analysis of generalized linear models in the presence of unmeasured confounding with applications to epidemiological research. *Statistics in Medicine*, 27(9):1539–1556. (Cited on page 147.)

Kamat, M. A., Blackshaw, J. A., Young, R., et al. 2019. PhenoScanner V2: an expanded tool for searching human genotype–phenotype associations. *Bioinformatics*, 35(22):4851–4853. (Cited on page 79.)

Kamstrup, P., Tybjaerg-Hansen, A., Steffensen, R., and Nordestgaard, B. 2009. Genetically elevated lipoprotein(a) and increased risk of myocardial infarction. *Journal of the American Medical Association*, 301(22):2331–2339. (Cited on pages 10 and 89.)

Kang, H., Jiang, Y., Zhao, Q., and Small, D. S. 2020. ivmodel: an R package for inference and sensitivity analysis of instrumental variables models with one endogenous variable. *arXiv*, 2002.08457. (Cited on page 129.)

Kang, H., Zhang, A., Cai, T., and Small, D. 2016. Instrumental variables estimation with some invalid instruments, and its application to Mendelian randomisation. *Journal of the American Statistical Association*, 111(513):132–144. (Cited on page 109.)

Kaptoge, S., Di Angelantonio, E., Lowe, G. et al. (Emerging Risk Factors Collaboration) 2010. C-reactive protein concentration and risk of coronary heart disease, stroke, and mortality: an individual participant meta-analysis. *The Lancet*, 375(9709):132–140. (Cited on page 7.)

Keavney, B., Danesh, J., Parish, S., et al. 2006. Fibrinogen and coronary heart disease: test of causality by 'Mendelian randomization'. *International Journal of Epidemiology*, 35(4):935–943. (Cited on page 10.)

Khandaker, G. M., Zuber, V., Rees, J. M., et al. 2020. Shared mechanisms between coronary heart disease and depression: findings from a large UK general population-based cohort. *Molecular Psychiatry*, 25:1477–1486. (Cited on page 10.)

Khaw, K., Bingham, S., Welch, A., et al. 2001. Relation between plasma ascorbic acid and mortality in men and women in EPIC-Norfolk prospective study: a prospective population study. *The Lancet*, 357(9257):657–663. (Cited on page 4.)

Kivimäki, M., Lawlor, D., Davey Smith, G., et al. 2008. Does high C-reactive protein concentration increase atherosclerosis? The Whitehall II Study. *PLoS ONE*, 3(8):e3013. (Cited on page 10.)

Labrecque, J. A. and Swanson, S. A. 2019. Interpretation and potential biases of Mendelian randomization estimates with time-varying exposures. *American Journal of Epidemiology*, 188(1):231–238. (Cited on page 139.)

Larsson, S. C., Bäck, M., Rees, J. M., Mason, A. M., and Burgess, S. 2020. Body mass index and body composition in relation to 14 cardiovascular conditions in UK Biobank: a Mendelian randomization study. *European Heart Journal*, 41(2):221–226. (Cited on page 150.)

Larsson, S. C., Burgess, S., and Michaëlsson, K. 2017a. Association of genetic variants related to serum calcium levels with coronary artery disease and myocardial infarction. *Journal of the American Medical Association*, 318(4):371–380. (Cited on page 10.)

Larsson, S. C., Traylor, M., Malik, R., Dichgans, M., Burgess, S., and Markus, H. S. 2017b. Modifiable pathways in Alzheimer's disease: Mendelian randomisation analysis. *British Medical Journal*, 359:j5375. (Cited on pages 10 and 170.)

Law, M., Morris, J., and Wald, N. 2009. Use of blood pressure lowering drugs in the prevention of cardiovascular disease: meta-analysis of 147 randomised trials in the context of expectations from prospective epidemiological studies. *British Medical Journal*, 338:b1665. (Cited on page 89.)

Law, M., Wald, N., and Rudnicka, A. 2003. Quantifying effect of statins on low density lipoprotein cholesterol, ischaemic heart disease, and stroke: systematic review and meta-analysis. *British Medical Journal*, 326(7404):1423. (Cited on page 89.)

Lawlor, D., Harbord, R., Sterne, J., Timpson, N., and Davey Smith, G. 2008. Mendelian randomization: using genes as instruments for making causal inferences in epidemiology. *Statistics in Medicine*, 27(8):1133–1163. (Cited on pages 20, 21, and 58.)

Lawlor, D. A., Tilling, K., and Davey Smith, G. 2016. Triangulation in aetiological epidemiology. *International Journal of Epidemiology*, 45(6):1866–1886. (Cited on pages 182 and 188.)

Lewis, S. and Davey Smith, G. 2005. Alcohol, ALDH2, and esophageal cancer: a meta-analysis which illustrates the potentials and limitations of a Mendelian randomization approach. *Cancer Epidemiology Biomarkers & Prevention*, 14(8):1967–1971. (Cited on pages 24, 135, and 136.)

Lewis, S. J., Zuccolo, L., Davey Smith, G., et al. 2012. Fetal alcohol exposure and IQ at age 8: evidence from a population-based birth-cohort study. *PLOS One*, 7(11):e49407. (Cited on page 10.)

Lincoff, A. M., Nicholls, S. J., Riesmeyer, J. S., et al. 2017. Evacetrapib and cardiovascular outcomes in high-risk vascular disease. *New England Journal of Medicine*, 376(20):1933–1942. (Cited on page 102.)

Liu, J. Z., Erlich, Y., and Pickrell, J. K. 2017. Case–control association mapping by proxy using family history of disease. *Nature Genetics*, 49(3):325–331. (Cited on page 191.)

Locke, A. E., Kahali, B., Berndt, S. I., et al. 2015. Genetic studies of body mass index yield new insights for obesity biology. *Nature*, 518(7538):197–206. (Cited on page 80.)

Lotta, L. A., Sharp, S. J., Burgess, S., et al. 2016. Association between low-density lipoprotein cholesterol–lowering genetic variants and risk of type 2 diabetes: a meta-analysis. *JAMA: Journal of the American Medical Association*, 316(13):1383–1391. (Cited on page 190.)

Maldonado, G. and Greenland, S. 2002. Estimating causal effects. *International Journal of Epidemiology*, 31(2):422–429. (Cited on page 28.)

Martens, E., Pestman, W., de Boer, A., Belitser, S., and Klungel, O. 2006. Instrumental variables: application and limitations. *Epidemiology*, 17(3):260–267. (Cited on page 16.)

Martinussen, T., Vansteelandt, S., Tchetgen Tchetgen, E. J., and Zucker, D. M. 2017. Instrumental variables estimation of exposure effects on a time-to-event endpoint using structural cumulative survival models. *Biometrics*, 73(4):1140–1149. (Cited on page 140.)

McPherson, J., et al. (The International Human Genome Mapping Consortium) 2001. A physical map of the human genome. *Nature*, 409(6822):934–941. (Cited on page 5.)

Mendel, G. 1866. Versuche über Pflanzen-hybriden. *Verhandlungen des naturforschenden Vereines in Brünn [Proceedings of the Natural History Society of Brünn]*, 4:3–47. (Cited on page 5.)

Mikusheva, A. 2010. Robust confidence sets in the presence of weak instruments. *Journal of Econometrics*, 157(2):236–247. (Cited on page 129.)

Mikusheva, A. and Poi, B. 2006. Tests and confidence sets with correct size when instruments are potentially weak. *Stata Journal*, 6(3):335–347. (Cited on page 129.)

Millard, L. A., Davies, N. M., Tilling, K., Gaunt, T. R., and Davey Smith, G. 2019. Searching for the causal effects of body mass index in over 300 000 participants in UK Biobank, using Mendelian randomization. *PLOS Genetics*, 15(2):e1007951. (Cited on page 170.)

Minelli, C., Thompson, J., Tobin, M., and Abrams, K. 2004. An integrated approach to the meta-analysis of genetic association studies using Mendelian randomization. *American Journal of Epidemiology*, 160(5):445–452. (Cited on pages 56 and 58.)

Minelli, C., van der Plaat, D. A., Leynaert, B., et al. 2018. Age at puberty and risk of asthma: A Mendelian randomisation study. *PLOS Medicine*, 15(8):e1002634. (Cited on pages 10 and 178.)

Minică, C. C., Dolan, C. V., Boomsma, D. I., de Geus, E., and Neale, M. C. 2018. Extending causality tests with genetic instruments: An integration of Mendelian randomization with the classical twin design. *Behavior Genetics*, 48(4):337–349. (Cited on page 191.)

Mokry, L. E., Ross, S., Ahmad, O. S., et al. 2015. Vitamin D and risk of multiple sclerosis: a Mendelian randomization study. *PLOS Medicine*, 12(8):e1001866. (Cited on pages 10, 84, and 173.)

Moreira, M. 2003. A conditional likelihood ratio test for structural models. *Econometrica*, 71(4):1027–1048. (Cited on pages 59 and 129.)

Mosteller, F. and Tukey, J. W. 1977. *Data analysis and regression: a second course in statistics*. Addison-Wesley Series in Behavioral Science: Quantitative Methods. (Cited on pages 109 and 116.)

Mountjoy, E., Davies, N. M., Plotnikov, D., et al. 2018. Education and myopia: assessing the direction of causality by mendelian randomisation. *British Medical Journal*, 361:k2022. (Cited on pages 10 and 164.)

Munafò, M. and Davey, S. G. 2018. Robust research needs many lines of evidence. *Nature*, 553(7689):399–401. (Cited on page 182.)

Nagar, A. 1959. The bias and moment matrix of the general k-class estimators of the parameters in simultaneous equations. *Econometrica: Journal of the Econometric Society*, 27(4):575–595. (Cited on page 132.)

Nazarzadeh, M., Pinho-Gomes, A.-C., Byrne, K. S., et al. 2019. Systolic blood pressure and risk of valvular heart disease: a Mendelian randomization study. *JAMA Cardiology*, 4(8):788–795. (Cited on page 10.)

Nelson, C. and Startz, R. 1990. The distribution of the instrumental variables estimator and its t-ratio when the instrument is a poor one. *Journal of Business*, 63(1):125–140. (Cited on page 122.)

Nitsch, D., Molokhia, M., Smeeth, L., DeStavola, B., Whittaker, J., and Leon, D. 2006. Limits to causal inference based on Mendelian randomization: a comparison with randomized controlled trials. *American Journal of Epidemiology*, 163(5):397–403. (Cited on page 17.)

O'Donoghue, M. L., Braunwald, E., White, H. D., et al. 2014. Effect of darapladib on major coronary events after an acute coronary syndrome: the SOLID-TIMI 52 randomized clinical trial. *Journal of the American Medical Associations*, 312(10):1006–1015. (Cited on page 43.)

Ogbuanu, I., Zhang, H., and Karmaus, W. 2009. Can we apply the Mendelian randomization methodology without considering epigenetic effects? *Emerging Themes in Epidemiology*, 6(1):3. (Cited on page 36.)

Palmer, T., Sterne, J., Harbord, R., et al. 2011a. Instrumental variable estimation of causal risk ratios and causal odds ratios in Mendelian randomization analyses. *American Journal of Epidemiology*, 173(12):1392–1403. (Cited on page 147.)

Palmer, T., Thompson, J., Tobin, M., Sheehan, N., and Burton, P. 2008. Adjusting for bias and unmeasured confounding in Mendelian randomization studies with binary responses. *International Journal of Epidemiology*, 37(5):1161–1168. (Cited on page 39.)

Palmer, T. M., Nordestgaard, B. G., Benn, M., et al. 2013. Association of plasma uric acid with ischaemic heart disease and blood pressure: Mendelian randomisation analysis of two large cohorts. *British Medical Journal*, 347:f4262. (Cited on page 178.)

Palmer, T. M., Ramsahai, R. R., Didelez, V., and Sheehan, N. A. 2011b. Nonparametric bounds for the causal effect in a binary instrumental-variable model. *The Stata Journal*, 11(3):345–367. (Cited on page 146.)

Patel, A., Burgess, S., Gill, D., and Newcombe, P. J. 2020. Inference with many correlated weak instruments and summary statistics. *arXiv*, 2005.01765. (Cited on page 143.)

Pauling, L., Itano, H., Singer, S., and Wells, I. 1949. Sickle cell anemia, a molecular disease. *Science*, 110(2865):543–548. (Cited on page 5.)

Pearl, J. 2000a. *Causality: models, reasoning, and inference*. Cambridge University Press. (Cited on pages 27 and 69.)

Pearl, J. 2000b. *Causality: models, reasoning, and inference. Chapter 3, Section 3.1: The back-door criterion*. Cambridge University Press. (Cited on page 30.)

Pearl, J. 2010. An introduction to causal inference. *The International Journal of Biostatistics*, 6(2):1–60. (Cited on page 28.)

Peto, R., Doll, R., Buckley, J., and Sporn, M. 1981. Can dietary beta-carotene materially reduce human cancer rates? *Nature*, 290:201–208. (Cited on page 4.)

Pierce, B. and Burgess, S. 2013. Efficient design for Mendelian randomization studies: subsample and two-sample instrumental variable estimators. *American Journal of Epidemiology*, 178(7):1177–1184. (Cited on page 129.)

Pierce, B. and VanderWeele, T. 2012. The effect of non-differential measurement error on bias, precision and power in Mendelian randomization studies. *International Journal of Epidemiology*, 41(5):1383–1393. (Cited on page 20.)

Plenge, R., Scolnick, E., and Altshuler, D. 2013. Validating therapeutic targets through human genetics. *Nature Reviews Drug Discovery*, 12(8):581–594. (Cited on page 93.)

Price, A. L., Patterson, N. J., Plenge, R. M., Weinblatt, M. E., Shadick, N. A., and Reich, D. 2006. Principal components analysis corrects for stratification in genome-wide association studies. *Nature Genetics*, 38(8):904–909. (Cited on page 137.)

Qi, G. and Chatterjee, N. 2019a. A comprehensive evaluation of methods for Mendelian randomization using realistic simulations of genome-wide association studies. *bioRxiv*, 702787. (Cited on page 117.)

Qi, G. and Chatterjee, N. 2019b. Mendelian randomization analysis using mixture models for robust and efficient estimation of causal effects. *Nature Communications*, 10:1941. (Cited on pages 105 and 115.)

R Development Core Team 2011. *R: A language and environment for statistical computing*. R Foundation for Statistical Computing, Vienna, Austria. (Cited on page 64.)

Rees, J. M., Foley, C. N., and Burgess, S. 2019a. Factorial Mendelian randomization: using genetic variants to assess interactions. *International Journal of Epidemiology*. (Cited on pages 160, 162, and 164.)

Rees, J. M., Wood, A. M., and Burgess, S. 2017. Extending the MR-Egger method for multivariable Mendelian randomization to correct for both measured and unmeasured pleiotropy. *Statistics in Medicine*, 36(29):4705–4718. (Cited on page 151.)

Rees, J. M., Wood, A. M., Dudbridge, F., and Burgess, S. 2019b. Robust methods in Mendelian randomization via penalization of heterogeneous causal estimates. *PLOS One*, 14(9):e0222362. (Cited on pages 75, 105, 108, and 109.)

Relton, C. and Davey Smith, G. 2012. Is epidemiology ready for epigenetics? *International Journal of Epidemiology*, 41(1):5–9. (Cited on page 189.)

Richardson, T. G., Sanderson, E., Elsworth, B., Tilling, K., and Davey Smith, G. 2020. Use of genetic variation to separate the effects of early and later life adiposity on disease risk: mendelian randomisation study. *British Medical Journal*, 369:m1203. (Cited on pages 140 and 154.)

Roberts, L., Davenport, R., Pennisi, E., and Marshall, E. 2001. A history of the Human Genome Project. *Science*, 291(5507):1195. (Cited on page 5.)

Robins, J. 1994. Correcting for non-compliance in randomized trials using structural nested mean models. *Communications in Statistics – Theory and Methods*, 23(8):2379–2412. (Cited on page 147.)

Robinson, J., Nedergaard, B., Rogers, W., et al. 2014. Effect of evolocumab or ezetimibe added to moderate-or high-intensity statin therapy on LDL-C lowering in patients with hypercholesterolemia: the LAPLACE-2 randomized clinical trial. *Journal of the American Medical Association*, 311(18):1870–1882. (Cited on page 94.)

Rossouw, J., et al. (Writing Group for the Women's Health Initiative Investigators) 2002. Risks and benefits of estrogen plus progestin in healthy postmenopausal women: principal results from the Women's Health Initiative randomized controlled trial. *Journal of the American Medical Association*, 288(3):321–333. (Cited on page 5.)

Rothwell, P. 2010. Commentary: External validity of results of randomized trials: disentangling a complex concept. *International Journal of Epidemiology*, 39(1):94–96. (Cited on page 83.)

Rubin, D. 1974. Estimating causal effects of treatments in randomized and nonrandomized studies. *Journal of Educational Psychology*, 66(5):688–701. (Cited on page 32.)

Rubin, D. 2008. For objective causal inference, design trumps analysis. *Annals of Applied Statistics*, 2(3):808–840. (Cited on page 192.)

Sabatine, M. S., Giugliano, R. P., Keech, A. C., et al. 2017. Evolocumab and clinical outcomes in patients with cardiovascular disease. *New England Journal of Medicine*, 376(18):1713–1722. (Cited on page 102.)

Sanderson, E., Davey Smith, G., Windmeijer, F., and Bowden, J. 2019. An examination of multivariable Mendelian randomization in the single sample and two-sample summary data settings. *International Journal of Epidemiology*, 48(3):713–727. (Cited on pages 150 and 152.)

Sanderson, E. and Windmeijer, F. 2016. A weak instrument F-test in linear IV models with multiple endogenous variables. *Journal of Econometrics*, 190(2):212–221. (Cited on page 152.)

Sarwar, N., Butterworth, A., Freitag, D., et al. (IL6R Genetics Consortium and Emerging Risk Factors Collaboration) 2012. Interleukin-6 receptor pathways in coronary heart disease: a collaborative meta-analysis of 82 studies. *Lancet*, 379(9822):1205–1213. (Cited on page 20.)

SAS (SAS Institute and SAS Publishing Staff) 2004. *SAS/STAT 9.1 User's Guide*. SAS Institute Inc, Cary, NC. (Cited on page 64.)

Schatzkin, A., Abnet, C., Cross, A., et al. 2009. Mendelian randomization: how it can – and cannot – help confirm causal relations between nutrition and cancer. *Cancer Prevention Research*, 2(2):104–113. (Cited on pages 24 and 85.)

Schmidt, A. F., Finan, C., Gordillo-Marañón, M., et al. 2020. Genetic drug target validation using Mendelian randomisation. *Nature Communications*, 11:3255. (Cited on page 142.)

Sheehan, N., Didelez, V., Burton, P., and Tobin, M. 2008. Mendelian randomisation and causal inference in observational epidemiology. *PLoS Medicine*, 5(8):e177. (Cited on page 20.)

Shendure, J. and Ji, H. 2008. Next-generation DNA sequencing. *Nature Biotechnology*, 26(10):1135–1145. (Cited on page 5.)

Slob, E. A. and Burgess, S. 2020. A comparison of robust Mendelian randomization methods using summary data. *Genetic Epidemiology*. (Cited on pages 108 and 117.)

Small, D. 2014. *ivpack: Instrumental variable estimation*. R package version 1.1. (Cited on page 65.)

Small, D. and Rosenbaum, P. 2008. War and wages: the strength of instrumental variables and their sensitivity to unobserved biases. *Journal of the American Statistical Association*, 103(483):924–933. (Cited on pages 129 and 188.)

Smith, J. G., Luk, K., Schulz, C.-A., et al. 2014. Association of low-density lipoprotein cholesterol–related genetic variants with aortic valve calcium and incident aortic stenosis. *Journal of the American Medical Association*, 312(17):1764–1771. (Cited on page 179.)

Solovieff, N., Cotsapas, C., Lee, P. H., Purcell, S. M., and Smoller, J. W. 2013. Pleiotropy in complex traits: challenges and strategies. *Nature Reviews Genetics*, 14(7):483–495. (Cited on page 179.)

Speliotes, E., Willer, C., Berndt, S., et al. 2010. Association analyses of 249,796 individuals reveal 18 new loci associated with body mass index. *Nature Genetics*, 42(11):937–948. (Cited on pages 80 and 156.)

Spiller, W., Davies, N. M., and Palmer, T. M. 2019. Software application profile: mrrobust – a tool for performing two-sample summary Mendelian randomization analyses. *International Journal of Epidemiology*, 48(3):684–690. (Cited on pages 79 and 119.)

Spirtes, P., Glymour, C., and Scheines, R. 2000. *Causation, prediction, and search*. MIT Press. (Cited on page 43.)

Stability Investigators 2014. Darapladib for preventing ischemic events in stable coronary heart disease. *New England Journal of Medicine*, 370(18):1702–1711. (Cited on page 43.)

Staiger, D. and Stock, J. 1997. Instrumental variables regression with weak instruments. *Econometrica*, 65(3):557–586. (Cited on page 124.)

Staley, J. R., Blackshaw, J., Kamat, M. A., et al. 2016. PhenoScanner: a database of human genotype-phenotype associations. *Bioinformatics*, 32(20):3207–3209. (Cited on page 79.)

Staley, J. R. and Burgess, S. 2017. Semiparametric methods for estimation of a nonlinear exposure-outcome relationship using instrumental variables with application to Mendelian randomization. *Genetic Epidemiology*, 41(4):341–352. (Cited on page 160.)

StataCorp 2009. *Stata Statistical Software: Release 11*. College Station, TX. (Cited on page 64.)

Sterne, J. and Davey Smith, G. 2001. Sifting the evidence – What's wrong with significance tests? *British Medical Journal*, 322:226–231. (Cited on page 95.)

Steyerberg, E., Bossuyt, P., and Lee, K. 2000. Clinical trials in acute myocardial infarction: Should we adjust for baseline characteristics? *American Heart Journal*, 139(5):745–751. (Cited on page 137.)

Stock, J. and Yogo, M. 2002. Testing for weak instruments in linear IV regression. *SSRN eLibrary*, 11:T0284. (Cited on page 129.)

Sudlow, C., Gallacher, J., Allen, N., et al. 2015. UK Biobank: an open access resource for identifying the causes of a wide range of complex diseases of middle and old age. *PLOS Medicine*, 12(3):e1001779. (Cited on page 63.)

Sun, L., Clarke, R., Bennett, D., et al. 2019a. Causal associations of blood lipids with risk of ischemic stroke and intracerebral hemorrhage in Chinese adults. *Nature Medicine*, 25(4):569–574. (Cited on page 190.)

Sun, Y.-Q., Burgess, S., Staley, J. R., et al. 2019b. Body mass index and all cause mortality in HUNT and UK Biobank studies: linear and non-linear mendelian randomisation analyses. *British Medical Journal*, 364:l1042. (Cited on pages 158 and 161.)

Sussman, J., Wood, R., and Hayward, R. 2010. An IV for the RCT: using instrumental variables to adjust for treatment contamination in randomised controlled trials. *British Medical Journal*, 340:c2073. (Cited on page 14.)

Swanson, S. A. and Hernán, M. A. 2013. Commentary: how to report instrumental variable analyses (suggestions welcome). *Epidemiology*, 24(3):370–374. (Cited on page 47.)

Swanson, S. A., Labrecque, J., and Hernán, M. A. 2018. Causal null hypotheses of sustained treatment strategies: What can be tested with an instrumental variable? *European Journal of Epidemiology*, 33(8):723–728. (Cited on pages 139 and 146.)

Swanson, S. A., Tiemeier, H., Ikram, M. A., and Hernán, M. A. 2017. Nature as a trialist?: Deconstructing the analogy between Mendelian randomization and randomized trials. *Epidemiology*, 28(5):653–659. (Cited on pages 139 and 183.)

Swerdlow, D., Holmes, M., Kuchenbaecker, K., et al. (The Interleukin-6 Receptor Mendelian Randomisation Analysis Consortium) 2012. The interleukin-6 receptor as a target for prevention of coronary heart disease: a Mendelian randomisation analysis. *Lancet*, 379(9822):1214–1224. (Cited on pages 20 and 40.)

Tardif, J.-C., Rhéaume, E., Lemieux Perreault, L.-P., et al. 2015. Pharmacogenomic determinants of the cardiovascular effects of dalcetrapib. *Circulation: Cardiovascular Genetics*, 8(2):372–382. (Cited on page 102.)

Taubes, G. and Mann, C. 1995. Epidemiology faces its limits. *Science*, 269(5221):164–169. (Cited on page 4.)

Taylor, A., Davies, N., Ware, J., VanderWeele, T., Davey Smith, G., and Munafò, M. 2014. Mendelian randomization in health research: Using appropriate genetic variants and avoiding biased estimates. *Economics & Human Biology*, 13:99–106. (Cited on page 133.)

Taylor, A. E., Richmond, R. C., Palviainen, T., et al. 2018. The effect of body mass index on smoking behaviour and nicotine metabolism: a Mendelian randomization study. *Human Molecular Genetics*, 28(8):1322–1330. (Cited on pages 64 and 165.)

Taylor, F., Ward, K., Moore, T., et al. 2013. Statins for the primary prevention of cardiovascular disease. *Cochrane Database of Systematic Reviews*, 2013:1. (Cited on page 88.)

Taylor, M., Tansey, K. E., Lawlor, D. A., et al. 2017. Testing the principles of Mendelian randomization: Opportunities and complications on a genomewide scale. *bioRxiv*, 124362. (Cited on page 18.)

Tchetgen Tchetgen, E., Walter, S., Vansteelandt, S., Martinussen, T., and Glymour, M. 2015. Instrumental variable estimation in a survival context. *Epidemiology*, 26(3):402–410. (Cited on page 140.)

Tchetgen Tchetgen, E. J., Sun, B., and Walter, S. 2017. The GENIUS approach to robust Mendelian randomization inference. *arXiv*, 1709.07779. (Cited on page 116.)

The Interleukin-1 Genetics Consortium 2015. Cardiometabolic consequences of genetic up-regulation of the interleukin-1 receptor antagonist: Mendelian randomisation analysis of more than one million individuals. *Lancet: Diabetes and Endocrinology*, 3(4):243–253. (Cited on pages 67, 68, and 190.)

The International Consortium for Blood Pressure Genome-Wide Association Studies 2011. Genetic variants in novel pathways influence blood pressure and cardiovascular disease risk. *Nature*, 478:103–109. (Cited on page 71.)

Thomas, D. and Conti, D. 2004. Commentary: the concept of 'Mendelian Randomization'. *International Journal of Epidemiology*, 33(1):21–25. (Cited on page 14.)

Thomas, D., Lawlor, D., and Thompson, J. 2007. Re: Estimation of bias in nongenetic observational studies using "Mendelian triangulation" by Bautista et al. *Annals of Epidemiology*, 17(7):511–513. (Cited on page 57.)

Thompson, J. R., Minelli, C., Abrams, K., Tobin, M., and Riley, R. 2005. Meta-analysis of genetic studies using Mendelian randomization – a multivariate approach. *Statistics in Medicine*, 24(14):2241–2254. (Cited on page 87.)

Thompson, J. R., Minelli, C., and Fabiola Del Greco, M. 2016. Mendelian randomization using public data from genetic consortia. *The International Journal of Biostatistics*, 12(2):20150074. (Cited on page 72.)

Thompson, S. G. and Sharp, S. 1999. Explaining heterogeneity in meta-analysis: a comparison of methods. *Statistics in Medicine*, 18(20):2693–2708. (Cited on page 77.)

Tobacco and Genetics Consortium 2010. Genome-wide meta-analyses identify multiple loci associated with smoking behavior. *Nature Genetics*, 42(5):441–447. (Cited on page 80.)

Tobin, M., Minelli, C., Burton, P., and Thompson, J. 2004. Commentary: Development of Mendelian randomization: from hypothesis test to 'Mendelian deconfounding'. *International Journal of Epidemiology*, 33(1):26–29. (Cited on pages 16 and 42.)

van Kippersluis, H. and Rietveld, C. A. 2018. Pleiotropy-robust Mendelian randomization. *International Journal of Epidemiology*, 47(4):1279–1288. (Cited on page 180.)

VanderWeele, T. 2009. Concerning the consistency assumption in causal inference. *Epidemiology*, 20(6):880–883. (Cited on page 43.)

VanderWeele, T., Tchetgen Tchetgen, E., Cornelis, M., and Kraft, P. 2014. Methodological challenges in Mendelian randomization. *Epidemiology*, 25(3):427–435. (Cited on pages 95 and 170.)

Vansteelandt, S., Bekaert, M., and Claeskens, G. 2012. On model selection and model misspecification in causal inference. *Statistical Methods in Medical Research*, 21(1):7–30. (Cited on page 62.)

Vansteelandt, S., Bowden, J., Babanezhad, M., and Goetghebeur, E. 2011. On instrumental variables estimation of causal odds ratios. *Statistical Science*, 26(3):403–422. (Cited on pages 63 and 139.)

Verbanck, M., Chen, C.-Y., Neale, B., and Do, R. 2018. Detection of widespread horizontal pleiotropy in causal relationships inferred from Mendelian randomization between complex traits and diseases. *Nature Genetics*, 50(5):693–698. (Cited on pages 105 and 108.)

Verzilli, C., Shah, T., Casas, J., et al. 2008. Bayesian meta-analysis of genetic association studies with different sets of markers. *American Journal of Human Genetics*, 82(4):859–872. (Cited on page 72.)

Wald, A. 1940. The fitting of straight lines if both variables are subject to error. *Annals of Mathematical Statistics*, 11(3):284–300. (Cited on page 51.)

Walter, S., Kubzansky, L. D., Koenen, K. C., et al. 2015. Revisiting Mendelian randomization studies of the effect of body mass index on depression. *American Journal of Medical Genetics – Part B: Neuropsychiatric Genetics*, 168(2):108–115. (Cited on page 189.)

Wardle, J., Carnell, S., Haworth, C., Farooqi, I., O'Rahilly, S., and Plomin, R. 2008. Obesity associated genetic variation in *FTO* is associated with diminished satiety. *Journal of Clinical Endocrinology & Metabolism*, 93(9):3640–3643. (Cited on pages 33 and 85.)

Waterworth, D., Ricketts, S., Song, K., et al. 2010. Genetic variants influencing circulating lipid levels and risk of coronary artery disease. *Arteriosclerosis, Thrombosis, and Vascular Biology*, 30(11):2264–2276. (Cited on page 86.)

Watson, J. and Crick, F. 1953. Molecular structure of nucleic acids: a structure for deoxyribose nucleic acid. *Nature*, 171(4356):737–738. (Cited on page 5.)

Wehby, G., Ohsfeldt, R., and Murray, J. 2008. "Mendelian randomization" equals instrumental variable analysis with genetic instruments. *Statistics in Medicine*, 27(15):2745–2749. (Cited on page 14.)

White, J., Sofat, R., Hemani, G., et al. 2015. Plasma urate and coronary heart disease: Mendelian randomisation analysis. *Lancet Diabetes & Endocrinology*, 4:327–336. (Cited on page 10.)

Willett, W. 1989. An overview of issues related to the correction of non-differential exposure measurement error in epidemiologic studies. *Statistics in Medicine*, 8(9):1031–1040. (Cited on page 123.)

Windmeijer, F., Farbmacher, H., Davies, N., and Davey Smith, G. 2018. On the use of the lasso for instrumental variables estimation with some invalid instruments. *Journal of the American Statistical Association*, 114(527):1339–1350. (Cited on page 109.)

Windmeijer, F., Liang, X., Hartwig, F. P., and Bowden, J. 2019. The confidence interval method for selecting valid instrumental variables. Technical report, University of Bristol, UK. (Cited on page 117.)

Wooldridge, J. 2009a. *Introductory econometrics: A modern approach. Chapter 15: Instrumental variables estimation and two stage least squares.* South-Western, Nashville, TN. (Cited on pages 62, 70, and 176.)

Wooldridge, J. 2009b. *Introductory econometrics: A modern approach. Chapter 5: Multiple regression analysis – OLS asymptotics.* South-Western, Nashville, TN. (Cited on page 141.)

Wright, P. 1928. *The tariff on animal and vegetable oils. Appendix B.* Macmillan, New York. (Cited on page 9.)

Yang, J., Ferreira, T., Morris, A., et al. 2012. Conditional and joint multiple-SNP analysis of GWAS summary statistics identifies additional variants influencing complex traits. *Nature Genetics*, 44(4):369–375. (Cited on page 142.)

Yavorska, O. O. and Burgess, S. 2017. MendelianRandomization: an R package for performing Mendelian randomization analyses using summarized data. *International Journal of Epidemiology*, 46(6):1734–1739. (Cited on pages 78, 119, and 152.)

Youngman, L., Keavney, B., Palmer, A., et al. 2000. Plasma fibrinogen and fibrinogen genotypes in 4685 cases of myocardial infarction and in 6002 controls: test of causality by 'Mendelian randomization'. *Circulation*, 102(Suppl II):31–32. (Cited on page 9.)

Zacho, J., Tybjaerg-Hansen, A., Jensen, J., Grande, P., Sillesen, H., and Nordestgaard, B. 2008. Genetically elevated C-reactive protein and ischemic vascular disease. *New England Journal of Medicine*, 359(18):1897–1908. (Cited on page 126.)

Zhao, Q., Chen, Y., Wang, J., and Small, D. S. 2019. Powerful three-sample genome-wide design and robust statistical inference in summary-data Mendelian randomization. *International Journal of Epidemiology*, 48(5):1478–1492. (Cited on page 174.)

Zhao, Q., Wang, J., Bowden, J., and Small, D. S. 2018. Statistical inference in two-sample summary-data Mendelian randomization using robust adjusted profile score. *arXiv*, 1801.09652. (Cited on pages 105 and 116.)

Zheng, J., Haberland, V., Baird, D., et al. 2020. Phenome-wide Mendelian randomization mapping the influence of the plasma proteome on complex diseases. *Nature Genetics*, 52(10):1122–1131. (Cited on page 179.)

Zohoori, N. and Savitz, D. 1997. Econometric approaches to epidemiologic data: Relating endogeneity and unobserved heterogeneity to confounding. *Annals of Epidemiology*, 7(4):251–257. (Cited on page 60.)

Zuber, V., Colijn, J. M., Klaver, C., and Burgess, S. 2020. Selecting likely causal risk factors from high-throughput experiments using multivariable Mendelian randomization. *Nature Communications*, 11:29. (Cited on pages 154 and 189.)

Index